21 Days to Eating Better

Books in the 21-Day Series

21 Days to a Better Quiet Time with God, by Timothy Jones

21 Days to a Thrifty Lifestyle, by Mike Yorkey

21 Days to Better Family Entertainment, by Robert G. DeMoss Jr.

21 Days to Better Fitness, by Maggie Greenwood-Robinson

21 Days to Eating Better, by Gregory Jantz

21 Days to Enjoying Your Bible, by Todd Temple

21 Days to Financial Freedom, by Dan Benson

21 Days to Helping Your Child Learn, by Cheri Fuller

A Proven Plan
for Beginning
New Habits

21 Days to Eating Better

Gregory Jantz

Series Editor
Dan Benson

ZondervanPublishingHouse
Grand Rapids, Michigan

A Division of HarperCollinsPublishers

CONTENTS

Day 1: Food and Mood   7
Don't Let Your Mood Determine Your Food

Day 2: Power Principles for Lifestyle Change   13
Keys to Authentic Living

Day 3: Take Control of Your Environment   19
Discovering What's Safe and What's Not

Day 4: The Power of Accountability   25
*The Excitement of Engaging Life Fully
and Being Open to Change*

Day 5: Build a Strong Spiritual Foundation   31
Luke 6:49 Says It Best . . .

Day 6: Say Good-bye to Stress and Guilt   37
*Removing Past Negative Emotions from
Your Food Choices*

Day 7: Surefire Fortifiers to Prevent Relapses   43
*A Temporary Period in Which We Retest
Old Behavior or Habits*

Day 8: Make Exercise Fun Again   49
It's Time to Throw Out the Rules

Day 9: Affirmations to Empower the Weary Pilgrim   55
*Why You Should Tell Yourself What
Is Already True*

Day 10: Your Personal Guide to Vibrant Health   61
*Everything You Do Is a Factor in Your
New Approach Toward Food*

Day 11: Finally, a Body You Can Love   67
   Cherishing the "Temple" God Gave You

Day 12: But What Do I Eat in a Restaurant?   73
   Staying in Control in High-Risk Food
   Situations . . . for the Rest of Your Life

Day 13: Relationship Principles to Set You Free   79
   Strategies to Create and Maintain Healthy
   Relationships That Build Openness and Trust

Day 14: Dealing with the Temptations of Foods   85
   How to Face Temptation and Not Give In

Day 15: Develop an Action Plan for Stress   91
   Having a Weight Challenge Does Not
   Necessarily Result from a Lack of Willpower;
   It's Often a Response to Stress

Day 16: Defuse Biological Time Bombs   97
   Bringing Health to Your Immune System

Day 17: Damage Control for Binges   103
   Bringing Your Life Back into Focus

Day 18: Nurture a Heart of Hope   109
   Grateful People Nourish Themselves
   with God and Others

Day 19: The Dance of Sex and Weight   115
   "Sexy" Sells. But Does It Really Deliver?

Day 20: How to Win with Food   121
   Your Path to Permanent Weight Loss

Day 21: The Day You Turn Your Life Around   129
   The Celebration Has Just Begun

DAY 1

Food and Mood

Don't Let Your Mood Determine Your Food

W hat kind of food do you plan to feed your mind today?" I asked Christine.

"Well, good stuff, of course," she answered.

So I pressed a little harder. "Give me some examples."

Long pause. Then Christine stood up, went to the window in my office, looked out into the parking lot, and said, "I want to feed my mind with good things today—like lots of positive thoughts, maybe a good book, and a passage of Scripture. But I don't see the relationship between what I feed my mind and what I will feed my body."

She's not alone. Many of us believe our bodies are one thing and our minds another. But last time I checked, both are located in one highly concentrated location—in something called YOU!

Have you ever thought that your eating habits may have some relationship to how you think and feel about yourself?

You may be saying negative things about yourself, then go out eating and bingeing, assuming you just have this terrible *eating* problem. When, in fact, it may not be an eating problem at all but rather, a *thinking* problem. The greater challenge may be not what you are eating, but what may be eating you.

So today, Day 1, we'll take a look at how closely connected your thinking *about* food is to the actual eating of food.

THE POWER OF A THOUGHT

Thoughts are powerful. Our thinking produces changes in our feelings, which, in turn, set us up for all our behaviors. The Bible says that as a person thinks in his heart, so is he (see Prov. 23:7).

This is how we all live our lives, even though we may not think about it very much: *Thoughts → Feelings → Actions*. Keep this sequence in mind.

Let's play this out on two fronts: The negative and the positive.

For example, say we engage in a kind of negative *thinking* that says, *I'm not very smart. It seems like everyone else is more successful than I am. I'll probably just always muddle along.* Okay, if that's the approach, then what kinds of *feelings* might result from this negative thinking?

It might be something like *I'm not worthy. I don't feel I'm really ever quite good enough. People don't love me. If they did, I'd probably feel better about myself.*

By holding these negative thoughts and feelings about yourself, what kind of *behaviors* do you think you could expect? Maybe something like, *Since I don't have any friends, I guess I'll make food my friend. I'm overweight, and I already feel miserable enough about myself, so what's the value of eating properly?*

Now let's look at the flip side of this conversation you're having with yourself—the brighter, positive side. You start out by thinking, *I may not be perfect, but I'm starting to like who I am. I'm enjoying life—with all its tremendous challenges. I know God loves me. I'm not always happy, but I try to be joyful.*

Wow, what a difference. Now, what *feelings* might emerge from this kind of positive thinking? How about something like *I feel blessed by a family that loves me. I feel supported by people in general, and God has given me the energy to love and support them, too. I feel hurt sometimes, but I know it's not permanent.*

And the *actions* that might arise from these positive feelings? *Because I know that my body is the temple of God, I'm going to treat it with respect and honor. I promise to feed my body with nourishing food just as I fill my mind with good, healthy thoughts.*

BEWARE THE PITCH!

And then it happens. Just when everything was going fine, you sit down to enjoy an evening of television, and here come the commercials. You see a juicy cheeseburger—a cholesterol nightmare—being eaten by a famous athlete. Your taste buds are stimulated. You've just eaten dinner, so a cheeseburger's not an option—but it does make you want to reach for the quart of ice cream or the box of chocolates. *Stop right there.* You are allowing your mood—dictated by the sights, sounds, and emotion of a television commercial—to determine your food.

Hit back. Instead of reaching for that box of chocolate, you may want to fall to the floor and do five or ten push-ups, or go for a brisk walk around the block, or get on your stationary bike. Notice how much better you feel—on two fronts:

1. You didn't buy into the hype of the commercial, and
2. You have physically done yourself a huge favor. You refused to allow your mood to determine your choice of food. By

choosing to do something physical, you released those special chemicals—called endorphins—produced by the brain that bring on pleasure and a sense of well-being. Marathon people refer to this as the "runner's high." But you don't need to be a runner to experience their positive effects. However, you'll quickly discover that a little sweat *can* make your day.

I want to make sure here on Day 1 that you are starting to *think* your way to better eating habits. So take a few quiet minutes with a pen or pencil to answer the following questions:

1. What kind of "self-talk" do I engage in most of the time? Is it positive and uplifting? Or do I put myself down with "stinking thinking"?

   _____

   _____

2. Am I eating out of fear, anger, or guilt? Do these moods cause me to eat mindlessly, compulsively, with little or no thought of the consequences of my actions?

   _____

   _____

3. Am I wearing certain clothing to *hide* how I look? How does this make me feel? What mood does it put me in?

   _____

   _____

4. What do I really want for my life? Am I willing to change my *thinking*, which will alter my *feelings*, which will change my *behaviors*?

   _____

   _____

This is not a test, and I don't want you to give yourself a score. But I do hope you'll take your answers seriously, because they're part of your foundation for moving on to a life of better, healthier eating.

Remember, it takes 21 days to break a habit. So just as Rome wasn't built in a day—or, as the Chinese say, *An overweight person didn't get that way with one bite*—so it will be with you in your pursuit of better eating and a healthier life.

Great work on Day 1. Now, let's get ready to put into practice some of the most important things you can do to create a lifestyle of permanent physical, social, and spiritual balance, coming up in Day 2.

LESSON OF THE DAY

Don't let your mood determine your food.

DAY 2

Power Principles for Lifestyle Change

Keys to Authentic Living

Have you ever felt that some people have an unbelievable excitement for life—something you'd give your eyeteeth for? But until now it just hasn't worked out? Maybe that's how you feel as we begin Day 2 of our journey toward better eating. If so, then let's ask some questions that may help you come to an understanding of *why* you may be feeling this way. Remember, this is only Day 2, so don't expect too much too soon. (We who have obsessive or semi-obsessive natures want to understand it all *now*. But remember, we have 21 days together.) For starters, let's take a look at some principles that will help you begin to know yourself better—even as you begin to make better food choices during our time together.

DISCOVER YOUR PURPOSE IN LIFE

Have you determined your purpose for being on planet Earth? If it is just to take up space, then it won't really matter much what you do with your life. You'll just coast along, careening from wall to wall, hoping that things somehow will work out. But when you believe that God loves you and that he really has designed your body to be a sacred "temple" for the Holy Spirit, then the picture changes. Because if God has given you your purpose, then the excitement of life arises from filling in the details.

When you understand that God has a unique purpose for your life, then you will want to know how to live out that purpose on a consistent basis. God's Word says you do it by renewing your mind daily. By choosing to be conformed to the image of Christ. By putting the right fuel in your mind, spirit, and body—and this includes eating the right kinds of foods. Because when you feel better physically, your "temple" will perform better emotionally, mentally, and spiritually—a proven formula for healthy, long-term growth. Something else: When you live life with purpose, direction, and seek worthy goals, you will not be so easily upended when temptation comes your way. Instead of caving in, you can ask yourself: *How is this junk food I'm about to eat going to help me with my purpose in life?*

LEARN THE JOYS OF HEALTHY BOUNDARIES

Foreign countries have boundaries. States have boundaries. Fences in our own backyards create boundaries. Boundaries don't have to be unfriendly, but they *are* necessary for those times when we just don't need the world breathing down our necks.

Healthy boundaries keep toxic people (you know who they are: negative folks with little gray clouds that follow them wherever they go) away from the passionate life you want to live. Here's the bottom line: The less you allow an invasion of the heart-snatchers, the less poison you will take into your own system. Mentally, I'd like you to put up a "boundary crossing" sign to help remind you where people may have overstepped their privileges in the past—and may even continue to do so in the present. These may be well-meaning but negative family influences. It may be some form of emotional or physical abuse that you've allowed to rule your life, making you feel inadequate and causing you to look elsewhere for comfort. And often, *food* is the comforter. That's why it's also important to recognize the need for food boundaries. If you don't have them, the "poison" of eating the wrong kinds of foods will keep you out of control, make you overeat and even binge on food. Boundaries protect you. They help to maintain your self-esteem and your God-given value. We'll be expanding on this theme in upcoming chapters.

BELIEVE IN YOUR POSITIVE FUTURE (GOD DOES)

For I know the plans I have for you,' declares the LORD, 'plans to prosper you and not to harm you, plans to give you hope and a future' (Jer. 29:11).

What a comforting verse. God has plans for us—and hope, and a future. That's good news, and I want you to believe it from the top of your head to the soles of your feet. When we know—and choose to claim—our exciting, positive future, we then have a reason to practice self-care. We start treating our bodies with respect by giving them the fuel they need, by eating foods that nourish, prevent illness, and even heal. We no longer invite inappropriate outside influences (there's that boundary issue again) to walk all over us. So keep making the decision that for these 21 days you will believe (because it's true) God has great plans for you and your exciting future.

RECRUIT A MENTOR/COACH

Someone has said that we may not have come over on the same ship, but we're all in the same boat. And another of our many common features is that we all have a need for a relationship with someone who has the wisdom and love to serve as our mentor—our coach, even as I am your playing coach during these 21 days.

Here's what mentors do:

- Model a healthy lifestyle
- Boost our self-esteem
- Give us honest feedback to help us monitor our progress
- Challenge us to live our purpose and follow our passion
- Practice and encourage healthy boundaries
- Live without obsessive-compulsive behaviors and addictions
- Believe in our positive future; mentors encourage
- Help us by leading the way, even though they are not perfect—no one is, but they are "living out" what we are becoming

I encourage you to find your own mentor today—and you'll find him or her more quickly by practicing the next key to authentic living.

PRACTICE A DAILY PRAYER-DRIVEN LIFE

No matter how much we work toward our most cherished goals, our labor will go unrewarded unless it is blanketed in daily prayer to our heavenly Father.

How might you pray? Here are some areas I pray for each day—reminders to me that I'm stuck in my tracks without the guidance of a gracious God to help me find my way. So I ask you to join me as together we . . .

- pray for strength to live a courageous life
- pray for a thankful spirit—an attitude of gratitude
- pray for the wisdom and insight to eat the right kinds of foods
- pray for an awareness that God wants us to honor (respect) the body (temple) he has designed and created for effective living
- pray to consistently make better food choices—and for the development of better food habits—during these 21 days and in the great future that lies ahead

Here's something I want you to highlight: *Be body wise.* Tell yourself the truth about what you do with food. When we're wise, we don't deny; when we don't deny, we do not lie—to ourselves, to others, or to God.

To be "body wise" means to make it a priority to keep the "temple" clean. Imagine what a clean machine your body can be after 21 days of taking this program seriously. But remember, it *will* take 21 days. Not 21 hours, or 21 hopes and dreams. 21 days. And you're already on your way to a healing, healthy lifestyle. Congratulations.

Remember:

- Wisdom is not chasing a fad.
- Wisdom is not being obsessed with food.
- Wisdom is not procrastination.

On this second day together, let's remember that wisdom is living a life designed by God and driven by prayer. It is cultivated living. Seek this wisdom and prepare yourself for truly authentic living.

Now get ready to take some more positive steps toward assuming control of your environment—learning what is safe and what is not safe for you, the freedom-giving theme of Day 3.

LESSON OF THE DAY

Authentic living is the only life worth living.

Take Control of Your Environment

Discovering What's Safe and What's Not

Have you ever been in the wrong place at the wrong time, wondering how on earth you keep ending up where you really don't want to be? I'm raising *my* hand to that question, because that's where I used to live. My problem was that I used to blame others for my sorrowful condition—until the day I looked in the mirror and saw a guy who looked an awful lot like me.

Why do we put ourselves in places that are unsafe—especially as it relates to food? Let's look at the 4 "P"s to see if we can come up with some answers: *places, people, palates,* and *positioning.*

REMOVE UNSAFE TRIGGER "PLACES"

Many of us have specific places that become "triggers" for poor food behavior. Consider these examples:

- Certain restaurants—comfortable places, but the wrong kind of food. Be aware of these places. Ask yourself: "Will the food I'm going to eat there bring me closer to my new, better-eating goals?" If not, stay away!
- Certain people's homes—where we don't want to be impolite but secretly admit we go there because we will *have* to eat whatever is prepared, saying, *Hey, it's not my fault. She cooked the meal. I had to eat it. I had no choice.* Politely, turn down some invitations. Suggest a healthy meal elsewhere; or cook a more balanced meal yourself—and invite your friends to your place.
- Certain rooms in our own homes—where we may hide to eat, or be so surrounded with food we go out of control. (Remove "hidden" food. Establish a "quarantine" from those rooms. Just as a restricted area protects others from sickness, so this quarantine protects you from yourself.)
- Certain old "binge routes" we travel when driving—usually consciously, because we know we'll be hungry *and will just have to stop at a favorite place.* Again the excuse, *Gee, it's not my fault, I was hungry.* (Take another, perhaps unfamiliar route. Enjoy a healthy piece of fruit as you drive to help you keep from getting too hungry.)

Unless you identify and take action, these trigger places will encourage you to go on automatic pilot, making it easy for you to eat foods that are improper fuel for our bodies. If we are not aware they exist, they will continue to control us and keep setting us up to feel bad about ourselves.

CREATE DISTANCE FROM UNSAFE TRIGGER "PEOPLE"

Some are well-meaning, some are not. But "toxic trigger" people are all around us, and they will do their best to exert control over our emotions. Take this example. You work in an office where one person just loves to go out to eat lunch every day, and because you're polite, you join her and the rest of the gang. The trouble is that she always picks the place where they have cheesecake to die for, and heaping chocolate sundaes with whipped cream cascading over the edges that will give you enough sugar for a week.

What do you do? Keep going out to eat with this person? Do you continue to order huge desserts when you don't want anything at all?

It's tough, I admit. But it's not impolite to say *I'm just going to have a salad today.* Is it really necessary to let another person dictate how, when, and what you should eat? When we let others rule our emotions, we have little choice but to feel bad about ourselves. Here's a phrase to remember: *We are the ones who teach others how to treat us.* We teach them how to hurt us with words, actions, passive-aggression, and nonverbal behavior. Have you ever felt about two inches high just because someone looked at you a certain way? No need to feel that any longer.

So what will it be? Toxic people or nurturing people? Those who pressure us to make poor choices, or who cause us to stagnate and rot emotionally, are toxic people; those who encourage us to be free, make our own decisions, and who want us to be all we can be are the folks who nurture us—and are the people we want to be around. And we cannot get enough of those kinds of friends.

CHANGE UNSAFE TRIGGER "PALATES"

Taste and smell are powerful triggers for memories and activities from our past. If we aren't aware of their incredible influence over our food choices, we may maintain a relationship with certain foods that go all the way back to childhood—connections that are the most powerful of all.

I have been counseling a woman who had been bonded to chocolate ever since her father owned a candy store, and candy and sweets were what she practically lived on for years. We've now worked out a plan where she doesn't go near a candy store, and where she changes the TV channel immediately if desserts or "sweets" are advertised. The triggers to her still-unresolved past are too intense. She continues to act out her child's perception of reality *fifty years later.* And fifty years is too long to stay in any kind of bondage.

When we "feel" a certain way, we will automatically want (have a drive for) certain foods. The advertisers know this, don't they? Remember the ad that challenges, "Bet you can't eat just one." They're right. But unless we're aware of this trigger, there will *never* be such a thing as "just a little."

The solution? We need to stop playing mind games with ourselves. The first sentence to cut from our vocabulary? *I'll just have one.* Don't have *any.* Remember, you *can* recondition your palate if you'll give it time, and it will take at least 21 days to change some of your tastes. Okay, it'll probably take a little longer to develop a fondness for brussel sprouts. (Or as one client pleaded with me, "Please, can't I just dip them in chocolate?") But there are plenty of great veggies and other healthy foods that taste great—maybe not on the first day you try them, but hang in there. Before long they'll be your food of choice.

SAY GOOD-BYE TO UNSAFE TRIGGER "POSITIONING"

You may have heard the phrase, *If it is to be, it's up to me.* It's a helpful reminder that you really do have the power to change much of your environment and, with God's help, assume greater control of your life as you make the journey toward better eating habits. To do this means you will need to be aware of unsafe trigger "positioning"—that is, those situations where you simply find yourself, or put yourself—consciously or unconsciously—in certain "eating" situations. Here are some practical examples of how to remove unsafe triggers from positions of temptation.

- Put the ice-cream scoop out of sight and out of reach.
- Remove from your home as many environmental "cues" as possible (cookies, bags of potato chips, peanut butter, processed cheeses, candy, fattening recipes, and so forth).
- Determine not to eat while watching TV, or while reading.
- Make it a point to sit down while eating, rather than standing by the sink devouring food compulsively.
- Clean out and redesign the inside of your fridge so you immediately see good, healthy food—not soft drinks, snacks, and desserts—when you open its doors. We not only are what we eat, but we are also what we look at and drool over before we eat it.
- Become an active participant in changing your surroundings from a negative influence to that of a healthy, enjoyable eating lifestyle. If you remain passive, hoping that somehow your surroundings will change as if by magic, they never will. It's up to you to remove the "positioning" triggers that have kept you in food bondage for so long.

THOUGHTS FOR POSITIVE CHANGE

Here are four encouraging thoughts to help you change your environmental settings, starting today. I encourage you to repeat these statements until they are as regular as your breathing:

- I have a plan, and I know where my life is headed.
- I am a person of purpose. God has given me certain areas in which I am in charge and in control. I am purposeful in managing these.

- I experience the presence and power of God at all times.
- I am already making better food choices because they are my decisions to make. I am taking full responsibility for my environment.

We now know that progress is not the same as perfection, and so our only sensible choice is the progressive realization of our worthy goals—a better, healthier definition of success. With this as a foundation, let's move on to the practical message of Day 4—how to accelerate our progress during the 21 days together through becoming accountable to another.

LESSON OF THE DAY

If it is to be, it's up to me.

DAY 4

The Power of Accountability

The Excitement of Engaging Life Fully and Being Open to Change

Have you ever felt that you were letting other people determine what kind of a day you were going to have? If they were angry, you got angry; if they were happy, you jumped on the happy wagon. If they felt you should go back for seconds and thirds at the local all-you-can-eat diner, you felt you simply couldn't refuse. After all—you were just being sociable. *It wasn't your fault.*

But that's really no way to live, is it? When we are not accountable—responsible, answerable—for our own actions, we actually make the choice to live in fear and misery, even as we continue to get taken for a ride that leads to nowhere. But let's make one thing clear as we begin Day 4. Accountability is not about punishment, retribution, "keeping score," or needing to be in control.

However, accountability *is* . . .

- a decision to be focused
- a determination to take specific healthy action—without excuse or regret
- the desire to be the very best we can be
- a system or plan that has enormous positive ramifications
- the practice of vulnerability and honesty, being willing to tell the truth, and being willing to accept feedback—even when the truth may be uncomfortable

FIND TWO PEOPLE YOU TRUST

When we feel we are damaging the quality of our lives with destructive eating and exercise habits, this is usually our first awareness of a need to change and to begin taking better responsibility for our lives. But we're usually not strong enough to do it all alone. That's when we need the nonjudgmental caring of people who care about us. For just a moment, think of two people whom you feel you can trust. They must have no axes to grind and should be friends who are kind, honest, and who care very much about you. If you have trouble thinking of these two friends, keep thinking. I know they will come to mind.

The issue: Let's say your challenge is overeating or consistently eating the wrong kinds of foods. In confidence you share your concerns with your friends, and you ask them to be your "sounding boards" as you determine to make serious changes in your eating habits. This may seem risky, and it may well be. But there can be neither growth nor accountability without some form of risk.

As your coach, I want you to use this brief "emotional checklist" as you engage the companionship of those with whom you will share an important part of your life.

- You must trust your friends implicitly and choose to be accountable to them—which means telling them the truth at all times, allowing them to give you honest feedback.
- They must not be your "rescuers." You are not looking for codependents. You want honest feedback so *you* can make the decisions *you* need to make to eat more responsibly.
- This is not a "power play." Your friends have not been issued military uniforms so they can exercise authority over you. You and God are your sole authorities. Only as you become aware of the person God designed you to become will you give yourself the permission to be shaped into the person you want to be. Growing people are accountable people. Years ago, Barbra Streisand had a hit song titled "People," which suggested that the luckiest people in the world were those who need people and the friendships of others. That's because there can be give-and-take—something that will only happen when we're in an honest, loving relationship.

GUIDELINES FOR ACCOUNTABILITY

What I'm now about to share will work for you *if you are willing to take the time and be disciplined to make it work.* As you make this part of your 21-day program for better eating, I am confident that you will begin to see results almost immediately. Here are the guidelines . . .

- Pray for wisdom from the very start. Do not say you're willing to be accountable if you are not. Being accountable means *being open and willing to change.*
- Develop a spirit of healthy accountability that prompts spiritual growth. Accountability with a caring friend also turns you toward God as you understand that he is the true source of your strength.

- Pray a daily prayer of gratitude. You will feel a new freedom, and you'll discover the rewards that come to you when you are courageous—that wonderful sense of well-being you get because you're finally taking full responsibility for how you are living your life.
- Deal with those *toxic secrets* that have kept you in bondage to unhealthy eating habits until now. You've chosen the road of responsible living by being vulnerable to people you can trust.
- Start keeping a log of your daily activities ... in 15-minute segments. Do this for the next several days of our 21-day program. This will take some discipline, but it will be worth it. You'll be writing a personal report card on what you are doing, what you are thinking, for what you are grateful, and whether or not you're accepting personal responsibility for your daily actions. Whenever I do this, I am amazed at how I'm actually living my life—even surprised, often, at how I may have lived the past hour. This activity always reminds me of Socrates' words, that "the unexamined life is not worth living." The Greek philosopher was right.
- Plan your accountability around specific issues—not just everything and anything that comes to mind. For example, you may want your friends to give you feedback on your eating habits at breakfast, or if you eat while watching television, or how you're doing on your new "activity" program. Choose specific events and then tune your ears to what your friends have to say to you.
- Make your accountability fun. Make it truthful. If you blow it, that's okay. Remember, you're after progress, not perfection. And have a good laugh if you go off the wagon and mess up royally. But after the laugh, look at your behavior seriously, because, in the end, it may not be a laughing matter.

- After approximately one month of being accountable to your two friends, consider transferring your individual accountability to a group. Being accountable to several people—the right group of people—will help you move from isolation to interdependency. It may be a self-help group, a 12-step program, a covenant group at church, or any number of healthy support networks. By sharing your progress with others, you will increase your self-confidence as you talk about your struggles honestly with fellow pilgrims. And together you will grow. Why? Because accountable people are growing people. They take full responsibility for their lives, and when they start to see the results, they are never the same.

I admit that Day 4 has been rather heavy, but to take responsibility for our relationship to food is no light issue. That's why we need each other in this pilgrimage. We were never meant to be islands of despair adrift in a sea of confusion. That's why I encourage you to find those two people who will be your friends to help you keep growing by keeping you accountable—an exercise that will help you build an emotionally strong foundation to help you think more appropriately about food—a theme we turn to in Day 5.

LESSON OF THE DAY

We are not islands. Accountability demands the courage to share who we are with others.

DAY 5

Build a Strong Spiritual Foundation

Luke 6:49 Says It Best . . .

But the one who hears my words and does not put them into practice is like a man who built a house on the ground without a foundation. The moment the torrent struck that house, it collapsed and its destruction was complete.

The preachers in the first century could hardly get used to the wonder of the Gospel, nor to the extraordinary composition of the church. It was so different from anything they'd ever seen. In that pagan culture, men and women crowded into fellowships for respite from their decaying society, seeking salvation as well as mental and social security. More than anything else, they wanted to belong. Without that fellowship, there was a sense of being orphaned, cut off, left in a cold, bleak desert of spiritual loneliness. Their own foundation had crumbled, and now, in the Gospel, they saw stability and a reason to live.

NURTURE VERSUS FORCE

Have you noticed how the best-laid plans, without a strong spiritual foundation, will often crumble? It was true in the early church; it is true for you and me today. Now that we've arrived at Day 5, let's take a look at the spiritual foundation that must be laid for *our* lives when it comes to how we treat the food we put into our bodies—the living temples of a holy, living God.

What does a spiritual foundation have to do with weight management and learning to eat better? I suppose the most important factor is simply to recognize that our bodies are the temples of God. They are not the "shacks" of God, or the "run-down dwellings" of God—but temples. Temples are to be treated with respect and honor. And that's how I want you to see yourself as we move through these 21 days: someone of great, immeasurable worth.

The next sentence contains the key to Day 5. Rather than force spiritual growth on ourselves, we will always treat our bodies and minds with greater respect when we nurture them through gentle development, thus creating a natural thirst for God's presence in our lives. Only then will we be free to hear his words of comfort and grace.

This nurturing begins with building a solid foundation. When the base is strong, the house will be stable. Then, as brick is placed upon brick (each a part of our whole person) the greater structure takes shape. These bricks must not be laid all at once—but one at a time and with great care.

DEVELOP A SPIRITUAL FOUNDATION OF SELF-CARE

As you move toward building a strong body free from an inappropriate love for food and food dependency, I encourage you to practice the presence of God in six key areas of your life . . .

- *Pray prayers of thanksgiving, petition, and praise.* A young boy, just learning to pray, said to his parents, "I'm going to pray now, and I'm going to be thankful. But, by the way, while I'm talking to God, do you need anything?" It's that kind of faith that moves mountains, and I encourage you to pray sincere prayers of gratitude to God for your blessings. The tragedy of our day will never be unanswered prayer but unoffered prayer—especially prayers of thanksgiving for that which we already have.

- *Reaching out versus reaching in.* The famous psychiatrist Karl Menninger said that generous people are rarely mentally ill people. He also said that love *cures* people—both the ones who give love and those who receive it. I want you to believe that to reach out is to reach for health and that to stay inward only sets you up for isolation, depression, and a dependency on food as your source of solace and comfort.

- *Practice love, acceptance, and forgiveness.* The author Jerry Cook says, "Do you ever ask, 'Why are we saying the Apostles' Creed?' 'Why this hymn?' 'Why hymns at all?' 'What is the application of church life out in the street, and how can what we are doing inside affect what's going on out there?'" If the Gospel—the Good News that Jesus Christ came to give us life abundant—that's been recorded, and is now being displayed on the giant screens of our daily lives, is not one that loves, accepts, and forgives, it becomes little more than another tired religious philosophy—one that doesn't merit being taken seriously. And here's the interesting twist: The more we love, accept, and forgive ourselves, the more we will love, accept, and forgive others. And when we behave in this manner, we will find ourselves so focused on people that we begin to eliminate food as a primary and inappropriate source of fulfillment or comfort. Instead, we give it its proper position: body fuel and nourishment.

- *Pray before eating and after (even after snacks).* In all sincerity, thank God for food for what it is: sustenance—the stuff that keeps you and me going. Thank your heavenly Father daily for creating food that sustains and heals—and do this before and after eating. When this becomes your act of worship, you begin to see food for how it helps you, which can help prevent you from abusing it or substituting it for other unresolved areas in your life.

- *Celebrate your life and trust God for wisdom.* When we abuse and misuse food, we have little to celebrate. But when we ask and trust God for his wisdom and counsel in relationship to what we put *into* our bodies, he freely supplies what we need to know—both through his Word, and through the insights of others. This is especially true when we live as though we truly believe we are a temple created by God. That's when we will have reason to become chronic enthusiasts for life itself. Daily celebration of God's goodness to us adds life to our years as we understand that nothing truly great is ever achieved without great excitement and enthusiasm. One key to a joyous, daily celebration is to tell at least one other person each day how God is leading and directing your life. There's that accountability issue again. If God is working in you, pass the good news on to others. It's a critical "brick" that needs to be laid in your spiritual foundation.

- *Recognize that a strong spiritual foundation is characterized by:*
  —A daily attitude of gratitude
  —A spirit of courage
  —The practice of patience
  —The joys of self-discipline

You and I are not perfect, and that's why gratitude, courage, patience, and self-discipline must be regarded as lifelong pursuits. Our goal must be progress, not perfection. We simply need to take baby steps in the direction of better self-care, better eating, better thinking about ourselves, and the building of a stronger, more solid foundation of spiritual principles, without which our house will be one built on sand and sure to be blown away by the first oncoming storm.

As you put these thoughts and ideas to work in your daily life, you strengthen your relationship with God, with food, and with those around you.

In a cartoon, the loan officer is talking to a person who wants a bank loan. He says to the prospective client, "We'll need more collateral than the fact that you expect to inherit the earth." Such a sentiment won't be enough to get us a loan at the bank, but it *is* what you and I have been promised as children of the King . . . and it's something we do not need to feel stressed or guilty about—as we'll see in Day 6.

LESSON OF THE DAY

Solid foundation first;
life abundant to follow.

DAY 6

Say Good-bye to Stress and Guilt

Removing Past Negative Emotions from Your Food Choices

How would you like to have a problem-free life? The kids never scream, the car never breaks down, the credit cards are never maxed out, and your relationships are always in top-notch condition? Sounds great, doesn't it? But you know what? It's never going to happen—not even if you do everything right for 21 days, or 210 days. Life is going to continue to be *life*. And with that daily living there is going to be stress, and yes, even some guilt for feeling we didn't do certain things just right.

So, you may ask, why do we have the word *good-bye* in the title for Day 6 if we'll never be able to rid ourselves of these twin pests? Here's why. When you say good-bye to your spouse as he or she leaves for work, or to your children when they go to school, or to a colleague at the end of a day, it's not good-bye for ever. It's only for a few hours—in some cases only a few minutes. You will be back. And the next day, you'll say good-bye again.

We use good-bye in Day 6 in this same way. Saying good-bye doesn't mean that our attitudes toward food and old food habits won't keep rearing their unsightly heads (although they should diminish over time), but it does mean we are starting to let go of enough old, unhealthy eating habits so that we do not perpetuate our toxic relationships with food.

STRESS AND GUILT

To have stress means that we're alive. If there were no stress in our fingers or wrists when we drink a glass of water, the glass would fall to the ground. But picture this: What if we remained in that "holding a glass" position all day—but holding no glass? Just pretending. That lack of motion would eventually take its toll on our entire body. Stress, in itself, is life and movement. We can't live without it.

But here's the problem. Inappropriate stress (stress that has little or no redeeming value) can lead to burnout, which can lead to emotional exhaustion. And from emotional exhaustion, it's only a short, bumpy ride to feeling unhappy, depressed, obsessive-compulsive, and then on to feelings of guilt for somehow having "missed the boat."

Authentic guilt is important for emotional growth. If you hurt someone and it's your fault, real guilt needs to set in, do its work, and then disappear. You do something about it, and you move on. The destructive thing we often do to ourselves, however, is to heap false guilt over our already tortured bodies, souls, and spirits. We are not wise to take on this kind of guilt, because really, it's not ours. And much of this false guilt has to do with our relationship to food. Diets, especially, teach us to be guilty, because there can be only one result: failure—and more stress. Diets don't work. Diets win. We lose. Every time. We buy the lie—hook, line, and sinker. So the question we need to ask ourselves is, *How long do I want to live under the pain of false guilt?* I hope your answer is, *Not much longer.*

If that is your answer, then you are going to make great progress on Day 6. Our goal today is to help give you a more stable framework for a stress-resistant, guilt-free relationship with food—where you no longer feel stressed or bad emotionally because of past eating habits. Here's a key point: *Your relationship with the foods you eat will either enhance your sense of well-being or it will promote shame and/or guilt.* Let's work at spotting some of these false trips before they begin to do their damage. We'll start by approaching some of what I'm going to call our "guilt" foods. Let's begin by doing a little exercise.

THREE HEALING THOUGHTS

1. Itemize four of your "guilt" foods. Ask yourself, "Why do I feel stressed and guilty when I eat _____, _____, _____, _____?"

In your mind, have you labeled any of these foods as "bad"? If so, who told you they were bad? How long ago? Was it your choice, or someone else's? Instead of thinking of these—or any foods, for that matter—as intrinsically good or bad, just ask yourself: *Are these foods contributing to my health and well being? Are they good for me?* I'll confess that I struggled with this battle for years because for much of my early life I had labeled many foods as "bad." The trouble with this was that when I ate these "bad foods," I also chose to believe that I was bad. I don't do this anymore, and you don't need to, either. I want you to know that there is no correlation between the two. A food may be good or bad for you, but neither one makes *you* bad or good.

2. Once you've re-framed foods into "healthy" and not-so-healthy, then you are ready for some real excitement,

because you are now going to give yourself a HUGE reward for improving your food choices. You will have renewed self-confidence because you are making conscious choices, something you may not have done until now. You're beginning to ask yourself questions, and you are no longer a victim of past programming.

You'll also find yourself with increasing amounts of energy. You'll start feeling healthier in both body and spirit. And you may discover that because you've begun to treat yourself with greater respect, your relationships with God and those you love will move to a new dimension. Because, when you begin to feel better, you'll want to be a better friend, a better spouse, a better worker, a better lover. What you feel about food has an immediate transfer to how you will feel about yourself.

3. When you are faced with a food choice in either a private or social setting, you now have the awareness and, I hope, the heartfelt desire to make a healthy food choice.

Let's take a quick quiz. Place the following foods into one of two categories: *Poor Choice* or *Healthy Choice*. Just put a √ in the column that best describes how you feel about that particular food. (Feel free to add to the list.)

Food	Poor Choice	Healthy Choice
Tomatoes		
Jelly donuts		
Steak		
Chips and salsa		
Ice cream		
Lettuce		
French fries		
Whole Milk		
Processed meats		

Food	Poor Choice	Healthy Choice
Salad with rich dressing		
Salad with lemon wedges		
Fried chicken		
Broiled fish		
Yogurt		
Cheeseburger		
Broccoli		
Tacos		
Cabbage		

AFFIRMATIONS FOR HEALTH

What does the above list look like to you? Do you think it will help you make healthier food choices during the next 21 days? Does seeing your choice in "black and white" help you see how you can put yourself in control of your choices? One of the best ways to help you stay on track is through the influence of repeated affirmations. Here is one I want you to recite aloud now—and repeat often . . .

I know what is best for my body, and I am taking full responsibility for choosing the right kind of food fuel to put in my tank. I am using my God-given common sense each time I eat. I have the freedom to choose foods that are good for me, or foods that are not. As with everything in life, whatever I choose is what I get to live with. For me, it's the healthy choice from now on.

From this day forward, I want you to do your best to keep your food choices healthy and simple. You'll be able to do this if you remember *that the food you eat is fuel,* not a convenient vehicle for the temporary resolution of unresolved emotional issues. Food is for the nourishment and sustenance of your mind and body.

As you see food in this new light—fuel for nourishment—for the next 21 days, you will begin to distance yourself from the former stress and the guilt that has kept you from making healthy food choices. Will it take time for your new awareness fully to take hold? Yes, about 21 days, amazingly enough. Is it worth the effort? I know what the answer is for me. And I'm praying that it's the same answer you've come up with.

It may not be Lent when you read this, but I hope you'll decide to give up stress and guilt as a bad deal anyway. If you have generally overeaten in response to being afraid, hurt, or in crisis, this would be an excellent time to develop a plan to help you eliminate your urge to overindulge when life's troubles begin to bog you down. Think of some ways you can respond to a typical challenge in your life so that you will not respond by "emotional eating." When you do this, you'll be making necessary preparation for the important "prevention" message you're about to read in Day 7.

LESSON OF THE DAY

I'm learning to make healthy food choices—and no longer identify myself with the foods I eat or have eaten.

DAY 7

Surefire Fortifiers to Prevent Relapses

A Temporary Period in Which We Retest Old Behavior or Habits

You may be saying, "Okay, I'm beginning to make some degree of progress here, and that's great. But how do I keep from slipping into my old, tried but untrue patterns of behavior? How do I keep my relapses to a minimum? Even avoid them all together?"

Good question. Important question. Relapses are a little like noses and ears: We all have them. But when we've been making progress and then suddenly relapse, we discover something amazing: *The old patterns don't quite work for us like they used to.*

Still, somehow we fool ourselves into thinking that our previous, threadbare behaviors will continue to help us—even though they did nothing but block our progress in the past. So we trot them out once again, thinking they'll work. But this is actually not all bad. Because this is exactly what happened to Linda.

THE PAYOFF'S NEVER WORTH IT

Linda was doing great with the new weight-awareness program we'd set up for her. Then she went off the wagon, ate everything in sight, hid great portions of food, and then sneaked away and ate it in the wee hours of the morning. In an instant, she began to live out her old bulimic pattern of behavior. Relapse!

It was not a good time for her. But, as it turned out, the relapse was such a terrible experience that Linda, in her own words, "came home" more quickly than she ever would have imagined.

What had once been a sick kind of pleasurable experience had now become mental and physical pain. The earlier "payoff" for Linda was no longer there. Instead, through self-discovery, she saw her situation differently now. She realized she was finally making progress *simply because her crisis had made her aware of what she was doing to herself, something she'd never been aware of before.* Relapses. We all have them—in many areas of our life. But why is it we relapse so much when it comes to food issues? (Anyone who has ever been on a diet knows the problem this is!)

I'm going to suggest at least two of the primary reasons why we tend to relapse into what we ultimately will admit is unproductive behavior:

- We relapse because we somehow forget that we have options, and
- We relapse out of anger, fear, stress, or rebellion, believing that our old, tired behaviors will once again give us control or power (even though they never helped us in the past).

FORTIFIERS TO GET US BACK ON TRACK

If you can identify with Linda, then it's time to exercise the following proven steps to prepare for a relapse before it blindsides you and destroys your hard-won self-confidence. If you work with these three preventives, you'll have less chance of setting yourself up for future failure.

GET LOTS OF REST

Rest and sleep are tremendous curatives for relapse. When I worked as a research aide at the University of Washington in our "sleep lab," we learned that when we're fatigued, we tend to eat more, eat less-healthy foods, and set ourselves up for depression.

This is why I want you to begin to reorganize your sleep patterns. Start to create nonrigid bedtimes for five nights a week—giving yourself no more than thirty minutes flexibility—either way—when you retire.

As you lie there, ready to sleep, take some time to thank God for each night he gives you to rest. As you thank your heavenly Father for his healing rest, you may want to think about the verse, "Therefore my heart is glad and my tongue rejoices; my body also will rest secure" (Ps. 16:9).

Start with a sleep goal of a minimum seven hours nightly. We now know that sleep patterns can be altered in as few as three days. Let your body go, and thank God in advance that he is blessing you with sleep. Your mind may still be racing for a while—and you may have trouble getting to sleep at first. But just follow your breathing and rest with a spirit of thankfulness.

Here's what will happen when you do this: Rest will equal renewal, which will begin to equal positive behavior. I encourage you to begin this pattern of resting and sleeping tonight. You'll be amazed at how, before long, you'll begin to stay on course with fewer food relapses.

LEARN TO RELAX

Relaxation is different from rest. It needs to happen during your busy day—when you *think* you have no time to relax. Actually you do, and it's one of the things you'll want to do each day during this program. Find a time to refocus, reenergize. It may be in prayer, meditation, or during your own special quiet time with God. Here's what I recommend: Allow yourself to be completely free from any interruptions for at least 15 minutes daily. There are several things you can do during this time. Here are a few:

- With your eyes closed, pray a psalm over and over—such as the Twenty-third Psalm. Actually "feel" the trees planted by the still waters. Actually "see" Jesus as your shepherd. Feel the Master take you into his arms. What a relaxing moment that can be.
- Breathe deeply and slowly as you feel the tension leave your body from the soles of your feet to the crown of your head. Do this over and over. Listen to your own breathing as you feel your entire body relax.
- If you are near a beach or can spend time in the mountains, don't bring a Walkman and a box of audiocassettes with you! Listen to the waves or the birds; feel the wind blow through your hair. Take time to enjoy God's great outdoors. It will be a tonic to your body and to your soul.

There are many wonderful ways to relax, but they will not happen automatically. You must make them a part of your daily schedule.

Give this practice at least ten days and you'll begin to see the benefits. By the time you have intentionally relaxed for 21 days, you will want to do it for the *rest* of your life. Relaxation is not a time waster. It is a time healer, and it will fortify you against tendencies to relapse into old behaviors.

RENEW OLD RELATIONSHIPS

Maintaining healthy relationships is a major secret to preventing relapses. In my experience in working with people over the years, I've discovered that each of us needs someone with whom we are fully accountable—like sponsors in AA. These are people who know us, accept us, love us, and who will be honest with us. One of your greatest fears may be the fear of "being known" by another. Yet, without facing this fear, you may be missing out on some of God's greatest blessings for your life.

As we become more intimate and vulnerable with others, we will begin to transfer what was once our intimacy with food to our new friendships. This will be a "relationship reminder" that the purpose of food is to nourish us, keep us healthy, and help us grow physically and emotionally, and not to be a quiet harbor to which we escape when we're depressed, angry, or out of control.

So if you feel that you are relapsing into rerun behaviors, I encourage you to pay serious attention to what's going on in your most immediate relationships. If you feel that a relapse is coming on, check out the status of your relationships for the past two or three days. Have they been healthy? Open? Free from frustrations? Where do you think you might have felt disconnected or isolated? Have your relationships been with "toxic," emotionally unsafe people? What you discover will give you many clues to your behavior.

RELATIONSHIP QUIZ

Here are a few important questions to ask yourself when reviewing the quality of your relationships:

- Who are the toxic people in my life?
- Who are my nurturing friends?
- To whom will I be truthful—even if it is difficult to be vulnerable?
- With whom do I have unresolved hurts? What am I prepared to do about this?
- Am I willing to become humble enough to forgive?

One of the most encouraging, faith-producing verses in the Bible is 2 Chronicles 7:14: "If my people, who are called by my name, will humble themselves and pray and seek my face and turn from their wicked ways, then will I hear from heaven and will forgive their sin and will heal their land."

You and I are able to forgive only because we have been forgiven.

When we keep our relationships clean, our emotions are cleansed.

When our relationships are healthy, we keep our relapses to a minimum.

As we exercise our spiritual muscles, we need to remember there are other muscles and joints and body parts that also need a working over. As we will learn in Day 8, the good news is that it won't cost much, and we don't need any special equipment.

LESSON OF THE DAY

Refreshing the soul is
the best medicine for relapses.

Make Exercise Fun Again

It's Time to Throw Out the Rules

John had just joined his fourth health club, but he still belonged to the other three. Never mind that he didn't use any of them. They were too old, he said, walls needed painting, equipment wasn't up-to-date enough, no juice bars, the trainers were just okay, and besides, parking wasn't all that terrific. John also had to walk too far from his car to get to the gym.

No one was more pleased than John when the new fitness center came to town. *Perhaps this one will do the trick*, he figured. *I'm not losing weight any place else, so it must be those other clubs. It can't be my fault. Finally, I've found a gym that just may work for me.*

Sound familiar? The *E* word: *ex-er-cise*. There, I said it!

But does it have to be so bad? Not at all. That's why in Day 8 we're going to help you make exercise fun again—a vital component in eating better, feeling better, and becoming the person God designed you to be.

For starters, what are the first three words that come to your mind when you think "exercise"? Write them down:

1. _____
2. _____
3. _____

Did you come up with "fun" words such as *Wow, excitement, can't wait?* Or did your mind race to expressions such as *dread, fear, competition,* or *no way!*? Whatever you wrote down, I want you to remember this: There are no rules.

The fitness centers of the world may not appreciate what I'm about to say, but here it is: Forget every rule you ever learned about exercise, because on Day 8 we're going to talk about exercise freedom—not pumping iron, running marathons, struggling to touch your toes (and ruining your lower back), sweating profusely, or feeling bad because you can't keep up with the gorillas in the gym. We're talking FREEDOM.

Consider these user-friendly guidelines for your exercise program:

1. I will not buy any special clothing or equipment to get started.
2. I will do nothing compulsively.
3. I will not engage in any obsessive exercise behavior.
4. I will simply make my body *move* in some way for a few minutes a day (even if it's putting golf balls on my carpet).
5. I will learn to enjoy my activity because I choose to do it.
6. I will engage in my exercise only because it is fun.
7. I will increase the amount of my activity only when *I* am ready to do so.

DO WHAT WORKS FOR YOU

Exercise must be something fully compatible with you and your personality. If you hate to run, don't run. (If you hate it, you won't do it, and so, why should you?) If a sweaty, inconvenient five-day-a-week regimen in a local fitness club is not for you, don't do it. That was John's problem. He'd conned himself to believe that he had to go for a big weight-loss program in a big club, with big fees, big trainers, and big, expensive equipment, or do nothing at all. Unfortunately, John chose nothing.

Exercise is not about feeling guilty for what you can't—or choose not to—do. The guiltier you feel, the less exercise you will engage in; and the less exercise you do, the guiltier you will feel, and your guilt cycle may produce so much depression, confusion, and anger that you may retreat to the "false comfort" of unhealthy eating again. The solution: Do what's right for you. Choose an activity that's *fun*.

YOU'VE GOT TWO LEGS—USE THEM

For many people, the best initial exercise program is simply to walk more. Walking requires no expensive club dues, no unique clothing, no special shoes, no time limits, no stopwatches, no subscriptions to fitness magazines, no nothing. It also burns calories and raises your heart rate. With walking there are also no excuses.

If it's hot, walk early. If it's raining, wear a raincoat or carry an umbrella, then come home and take a hot shower. (Note: If you live in Alaska or some other cold climate and it's winter and you can't walk without freezing, you might consider walking in place, or riding a stationary bike, or doing some push-ups, or bouncing for a few minutes each day on a small trampoline.)

NO EXCUSES, PLEASE

People who are serious about exercise and its relationship to better eating do not make excuses. They are realistic, and they make their activity program work for them. Exercise is their slave, not their master.

When they walk, they know it directs a hefty supply of oxygen to their brain (releasing endorphins, nature's own "mood" makers), lungs, and circulatory system, helps provide clarity of thinking, gives them a chance to be away from their busy life for a few moments, helps them think about their progress as they move toward permanent weight loss, provides a few moments to listen to the birds, smell the flowers, and to spend quality time talking with their spouse, a neighbor, or a friend as they take on the familiar and unfamiliar streets and lanes of their neighborhood.

DISMOUNT THE GUILT CYCLE

Here are some good questions to ask yourself: What do I really want in my life? Do I want a body to rival the latest cover girl on my favorite magazine, or do I want happiness and a deep sense of inner joy? Do I really want "buns of steel," or would I be happier with lasting peace of mind, good friends, and a trimmer shape as simple by-products of my exercise regimen?

You already know that unfulfilled expectations invariably lead to guilt, which leads to depression, which leads to compulsive behavior eating, which leads to using food for comfort—comfort to get out of the depression, which leads back to anger at ourselves that we *did it again!* This anger paralyzes us with the fear that we're never going to able to do this . . . and the beat goes on. So let's deal with this challenge head-on and put it to rest.

RESHAPE YOUR THINKING— AS WELL AS YOUR BODY

Positive self-talk has helped hundreds of the people who have come to me for counseling but only when repeated daily and put into active practice. The following are my special gifts to you on Day 8. As you say these statements to yourself, speak them with enthusiasm, excitement, and with reckless abandon—even if they are not actually a part of your thinking yet. I promise you they soon will be.

- God made me an active, alive human being. I am enthusiastically believing this truth as I enjoy my life to its fullest at all times.

- God made my body to move, not to sit still. That's why I engage in some form of exercise for at least ten to fifteen minutes a day. I am happy there are no rules for my activity, because this means I can never lose the game. I am determined to be active because I know I will then never rust out.

- I am excited about my balanced schedule of activity. I do what I can when I can do it. I feel good about myself just knowing that I'm going for progress, not perfection. I engage in my activity with joy and enthusiasm because I know it's these daily baby steps that bring me closer to my goal.

- I am increasing my activity level a little bit at a time, and I feel my body responding with a resounding *THANK YOU!*

- My attitude is my choice, and I choose to be active because I care about the body God has given me. It *is* a temple of God, and it deserves the best of everything. Nothing can stop me now. I am thrilled that I can enjoy my daily activity for its sheer enjoyment. I am choosing a healthy, positive attitude about my daily success. I feel great!

Well, what do you think? Has Day 8 been good to you? Are you ready to start making exercise fun again? I trust that the answer is YES. But just like anything in life that's worthwhile, you'll also have to exercise patience. It takes time to "believe"—remember, it takes 21 days to make or break a habit—that your smallest activity is essential to your long-range goals. But take it from your coach: It will be more than worth the effort, because before long, you'll find yourself filled with increased amounts of fresh, new, emotional, physical, and mental energy.

And one of the best exercises of all is the joy of affirming the truth about who we really are and saying goodbye to the lies we used to tell ourselves . . . the theme in Day 9 that just might change your life forever.

LESSON OF THE DAY

Exercise is all about freedom.

DAY 9

Affirmations to Empower the Weary Pilgrim

Why You Should Tell Yourself What Is Already True

To understand affirmations, it is first important to understand the opposite—those many "misbeliefs" we have about ourselves and our performance. While this is a serious subject, I think we'd all have to confess that we believe and say some pretty ridiculous things about ourselves on occasion. Things that bear little or no resemblance to reality.

For example, on the tennis court we may miss a ball and say, "Come on, you dummy, how come you missed such an easy shot?" Not true. A simple error in a recreational sport does not make you a dummy.

Or after a rough morning with the kids—and the hassle of getting them ready for school—you may say, "I just can't do anything right. I'm always making the same, stupid mistakes." Again, not true. You may have had a bad morning, but it's not a truthful statement that you "can't do anything right."

Or after working on disciplined eating—and feeling good about yourself for eating healthy foods—you suddenly binge for two days. With feelings of guilt and frustration you say, "I knew I couldn't do it. I knew I was weak. I guess I'll just never have a healthy body. I'll always be fat." Lies. Statements of misbelief. But so very powerful.

THE CAUSE: EMOTIONAL TURMOIL

The tragedy here is this: The more you and I speak—and repeat—such statements of misbelief, the more a perverse negativity invades our conscious and our unconscious minds, creating yet more negative, battered emotions, setting us up for more destructive behavior and sending us spiraling into confusion from which we may feel there is no escape.

Statements of misbelief arise primarily from emotional turmoil—where we've become so weary that we simply opt for the easy way out: *I'm no good. I'll never amount to anything. I'm overweight, and there's nothing I can do about it* . . . and the list of reasons to fail continues.

SAME ENERGY: DIFFERENT FOCUS

Okay, enough on the negative side. Here on Day 9, I want you to take the same heightened emotions of some of your misbelief statements and pour them into statements of belief in yourself. You need to believe in yourself to perform, accept, give, love, and be open and vulnerable. Remember that a strong belief in yourself is the most important endorsement you'll ever get. That's why daily, personal affirmations are so important: It is your private opportunity to tell yourself something that is already true! That's today's key statement. When we say good things about ourselves, we speak the truth. The challenge is to replace the lies we tell ourselves with this truth.

Misbeliefs about who we say we are are like pesky weeds. They grow without being planted, watered, or nurtured. They're just there. All the time. And if we don't weed them from the gardens of our minds, those troublesome weeds will just keep growing and growing.

Truth, however, spoken in the form of affirmations is like an old oak. Its roots go deep. It makes us better over time. It helps us weather the storms of life and makes us stronger.

FREE TO RISK, CHANGE, TRUST, LOVE

Affirmations make us *free to risk*. They help us let go of the past to live fully in the present (1 Peter 5:6–7).

Example: I see myself as a person of ideal weight. I am eating nutritious food, and I like the way my body feels. I am on my way to better eating habits.

Affirmations help us to be *free to change*. They permit us to be transformed from the inside out by the renewing of our minds (Rom. 12:2).

Example: I may not be what I want to become yet, but I'm also not where I once was. I am making measurable progress in reasonable time, and I believe that my body is the temple of God. I am making good food choices, and I am choosing to live a vibrant life.

Affirmations help us become *free to trust*. They freshen our perspective, help us to honor our heavenly Father, and help us understand why it is important to give him thanks for the way he made us (1 Cor. 6:19).

Example: I am glad God made me as I am. I know he has poured himself into me, and because of his bountiful gifts, I thank him and trust him. My new attitude is also helping me trust and be grateful for the many other blessings in my life.

Affirmations provide us with the wherewithal that helps us be *free to love and accept others and ourselves*. In a world of suspicion, jaded thinking, and doubt, affirmations give us the confidence and freedom to practice love, acceptance, and forgiveness (John 13:34).

Example: This is a special day for me. I have a choice to love others and to accept myself—and I happily accept myself just as I am today. With God's help, I am finding I'm able to love and forgive, and it is making a difference in my life.

WHAT YOU CAN EXPECT

How does it feel when you repeat these affirmations? Comfortable? Uncomfortable? However you *feel* about saying them, remember, *they are all statements of truth.* That's the singular idea I want you to capture here on Day 9. And as you learn to make these affirmations part of your life, here's what you'll start to experience. You will . . .

- choose to be bold with reality—not with what you *thought* was reality.
- begin to live your life as God designed you to live it.
- relieve yourself from unhealthy or improper guilt and shame.
- enjoy the freedom of expressing yourself—which will help enhance your self-esteem.
- discover that you really *do* have a future and a hope for better things to come.
- receive the best prescription possible for your recovery from obsessive-compulsive behaviors and unhealthy habits.
- begin, finally, to be honest with your feelings toward yourself, others, and to God.

YOUR TURN

On the following lines, I would like you to write three affirmations of your own. You also may want to write them out on 3 x

5 cards and carry them with you at all times. Here are the ground rules.

Keep them in the present tense—"I am, I see myself," and so forth.

Say them with great energy and emotion. After all, you are speaking the truth, and the truth must never be mumbled. Repeat your affirmations at least two times daily—you choose the times best suited for you. Most of my clients repeat theirs during breakfast and just before going to bed.

Choose those areas where you want to make measurable progress in reasonable time.

Remember: The fact that you have not yet achieved your goal does not negate your affirmation. The brain cannot differentiate between affirming a truth and the actual fact. That's why both a misbelief and an affirmation have equal power to rule our lives. Okay, now it's your turn . . .

THREE AFFIRMATIONS

1. _____
   _____
2. _____
   _____
3. _____
   _____

I wish I could see what you've written. Perhaps you'll be willing to share them with me. What you've just put on paper are building blocks of joy. They are the "industrial strength" cleansers you need for a pure (nontoxic) thought life. Your affirmations are helping you take a giant step toward building a fortress to insulate you from the destructive invasion of unhealthy thoughts and the negative actions of others.

THE BIBLE AS HOMEWORK

Here's a great idea. Open your Bible to the Psalms or the Proverbs and read several passages each day in an "affirmation mode." These verses will come to life and begin, almost, to jump off the page. God's Word will never be quite the same for you again.

You'll find yourself cleansing, rebuilding, and replacing your false thinking/misbeliefs with the truth. And when you do this consistently for 21 days, you will develop a spiritual and emotional foundation to help you face the challenges of life. I promise you, it works, and it will be a grand prelude to what you will discover in Day 10—your personal, practical guide to vibrant health.

LESSON OF THE DAY

To speak an affirmation is to tell myself what I know is true.

DAY 10

Your Personal Guide to Vibrant Health

*Everything You Do Is a Factor in Your
New Approach Toward Food*

I'll call her Sheila—not her real name. When she came to see me two years ago, she had done just about everything opposite to what we've learned from days 1 through 9. She had been allowing her mood to determine her food ("I can't help it, the TV commercial was all about pie and ice cream"); she was allowing people, places, and events to "trigger" her eating habits ("If Martha just wouldn't bake those chocolate cookies, I wouldn't be so fat"); and about the only exercise she got was jumping to conclusions and running other people down because they were so skinny—and probably malnourished.

The good news is that Sheila finally became sick and tired of being sick and tired—and overweight, and feeling lousy. That's when I put her on the program that we're going through during these 21 days together. And it really *did* take her about 21 days to grasp what it means to develop better eating habits.

Here's what she wrote to me after our last session together:

Dear Dr. Jantz,

I never thought I would feel this good. I know you must have thought, at times, that I was your most difficult client. But I've got to tell you that I have never felt better and have never been in such vibrant health—emotionally, spiritually, and physically. Exercise is fun again (I walked five miles today), and I gave my scale to the Salvation Army. You were right. Who needs scales? It's not about weight; it's about eating well and feeling good. Please use this brief note to encourage others if you so desire. Thanks again for helping me regain my life.

Your friend,
Sheila

If Sheila could learn to discipline herself to enjoy this kind of success, so can you. And Day 10 will take you that one confident step closer to enjoying abundant, vibrant health—the kind that God created you to enjoy.

Do you still remember our underlying theme for these 21 days?—that we're after progress, not perfection? Keep that in mind. Because with *major progress* comes *major self-confidence,* and *major success.* Let's look at five key ingredients for this exciting, vibrant life that lies just ahead for you.

ENJOY MORE HEALTHY ACTIVITIES

People like you, who are learning to eat better, are learning the value of choosing to be active as opposed to living a life of isolation. Unless you have a direct call from God, you were probably not destined to be a monk—isolated and out of touch. That's why I encourage you to become involved with a group of people who share your ideals and goals. It may be a Bible study, or helping seniors in their activities at a retirement home, or the fun of a weekend tennis or hiking group (but probably *not* a gourmet eating society—at least not yet).

When you become more active—physically, spiritually, and relationally—you'll have a better chance of disciplining yourself to turn your attention away from food and start focusing on people. As this happens, you will also begin to avoid extreme behaviors such as obsessive-compulsive eating and bingeing. And because of your increasingly active life, when you need a friend to help you in a crisis situation, you'll have people around you who care.

BELIEVE IN YOUR POSITIVE FUTURE

Those who practice telling themselves the truth on a daily basis are willing to look at faulty belief patterns (misbeliefs) and make corrections midcourse. This is the foundation for your better future. Does this mean that your life will be without problems from now on? No. But it is the basis for your honest-to-goodness, positive future. Does this mean that everything is going to come up roses? No. But you will become more aware of the roses around you than the thorns.

Here's a thought—and a definition—to help you put all this together: A "belief" is an acquired judgment that is useful only if it is open to change. If you *believe* it will rain today (and you've already promised yourself you will feel just awful if it does), then the rain is going to affect your mood. Here's the formula: A belief tells us how to *think*, which leads to how to *feel*, which tells us how to *act*. Here on Day 10, as you move a day closer to better eating habits, you are beginning to replace faulty, negative, destructive beliefs with true, positive, edifying beliefs. Your new belief system says, *I am in charge of the food I put in my mouth, instead of food being in charge of me.* And it all starts with what you choose to believe.

REVIVE YOUR SPIRITS DAILY

Let me ask you a question: *How tall will a tree grow?* Wouldn't you agree it will grow as tall as it's been designed by God to grow? Trees don't think limits. They just keep growing and growing, as if they didn't know better. Now that's how I want you to keep thinking about every aspect of your life during each of these 21 days. Don't think limits. Think *growth*. Think of the exciting possibilities that are ahead for you—and they may be around the next corner.

You have hundreds of choices each day—and food is one of them. You can choose nutritious food or lousy, unhealthful junk. It's up to you. But when you make healthy food choices, you are making life-giving choices that really do matter—especially as you keep in mind that your body (which includes your soul and spirit) is the temple of God. So how will you revive your spirits today: By making a new friend? Taking the time to listen to a child? Going on a great hike? Calling someone you haven't spoken to for 10 years? By asking someone's forgiveness? The possibilities are endless—so go at them with all the enthusiasm your heart can muster. You may ask what "reviving my spirits" has to do with eating better and developing a more appropriate view of food. It's all about seeing yourself as a *whole* person. Just as stones in a mosaic are vital to the entire picture, so does *everything you do have something to do with the rest of you.*

WORK ON YOUR RELATIONSHIPS

Again, think wholistically. Positive relationships are vital to turning your eating habits around. As you begin to develop better eating habits, you will start to put your emphasis on the development of healthy relationships, not on food. During each of these 21 days, you are increasingly giving yourself over to be used by God, as opposed to being controlled by an external source—in this case, food. This is because you are finally breaking the "cycle of indulgence" with food and are starting to see the importance of your relationships in a new light. You are now pushing yourself away from the table and moving closer to those you care about—those who need to be understood, accepted, and affirmed.

Close relationships with both men and women are essential to your progress during these 21 days. Remember that you are not an island. The feeling of attachment, of caring about someone, is what a vibrant life is all about. That's why I want you to keep taking day-by-day steps toward developing friendships and the joys that will come your way as a result of focusing on people, not food. It's all part of developing the "wholeness" of you.

DEVELOP A HEART OF WISDOM

Get wisdom, get understanding; do not forget my words or swerve from them," says the writer in Proverbs 4:5. With God's Word as our foundation, let's look at some levels of wisdom as they relate to food choices and vibrant health.

- *Common sense.* Most of the time you know what you should eat. It's obvious. When you look at a menu, you can choose a healthy light lunch of salad with lemon wedges and a couple of crackers, or a mouth-watering BLT with bacon, mayonnaise, and other sundry forms of grease that will soon be dripping from your chin. Stop and ask yourself, *What is the commonsense thing for me to eat at this time?*

- *The practical.* This is less obvious than common sense. It may not be practical to have "nuts and twigs" at the next dinner party you plan to host. But as you plan your menu, you *do* have the choice of what to serve. What will it be? Fattening foods that will keep your guests up all night, reaching for Rolaids? Or will you bless them with foods that are light, healthful, and life-giving? This may involve some risk. I realize that. But be bold and be confident. You may discover that exploring uncharted "food" territory is the talk of your party.

- *Discernment that's God-given and God-directed.* This wisdom will come when you ask for and seek God's will for your life. The more you cry out to God for his wisdom in all areas of your life—including your challenges with food—the more he will hear your cries and give you the insight you need. What wisdom do you need from the Father today? List 3 areas:

a. _____

b. _____

c. _____

Let's close Day 10 with this affirmation:

I choose to live a life filled with healthy activities, a positive belief in my better future, a daily, revived spirit, stronger relationships, and a fresh awareness of my need for wisdom. I know these ingredients will help me see my life as a *whole,* bringing me closer to my goal of a healthier, more vibrant life. This is my choice for each of these 21 days and for every day thereafter.

With that promise to yourself, fasten your seat belt, because Day 11 is going to place before you some powerful decisions you can make *right now* to help you develop a new appreciation for the physical body God has given you.

LESSON OF THE DAY

I'm preparing for life's future challenges by choosing to live a vibrant life today.

Finally, a Body You Can Love

Cherishing the "Temple" God Gave You

Okay, let's get the key questions out of the way in the first paragraph: *Do you like your body? Do you love your body? Is your body your friend?*

If you're like many of the people I work with, the answers are not long in coming. Most tell me, "You've got to be kidding. This body? No way!" Or, "I just read this month's copy of *Glamour* magazine, and you have the audacity to ask me if I like *my* body?" That's when I hold up a white flag (which I keep handy in my top drawer for just such occasions) and declare a truce before we even get started. Unless I miss my guess, you may be feeling the same way.

But here's the good news: On this eleventh day together, you really can learn to start to like—and yes, even love—your body. Even in its present shape, weight, and age. Now you may be saying, "Dr. Jantz, is this a course in denial, or what?" Actually, it's quite the opposite, as you'll soon see.

NAMES THAT HURT

First of all, we all have strong emotional feelings and opinions about our bodies, most of which come from our past. When you were a child, someone may have said, "Wow, will you look at that snozola!" or "Man! With those Dumbo ears, I bet she can fly!" Ouch. Those comments hurt then ... and they may continue to affect how you feel about your body now. Or you may have been heavier than the others in your junior high or high school, and some may have laughed at you, calling you such names as pig, or cow, or tub of lard. Or you may have been so skinny that you said to yourself, *Just you wait, I'll fatten up, and I'll show you.* And you did a good job of it. Too good a job, perhaps.

ABOUT THAT BODY

Let's do a quick survey to help you see how you relate to your own body. (After you've written your comments, circle each one with a 1 to 10. 1 = "I hate my body" to 10 = "I love my body.")

A. What two parts of your body have you always liked?
    1. _____ 2. _____
    To what degree? 1 2 3 4 5 6 7 8 9 10
B. What two areas of your body are sort of okay?
    1. _____ 2. _____
    To what degree? 1 2 3 4 5 6 7 8 9 10
C. What two areas of your body do you dislike intensely?
    1. _____ 2. _____
    To what degree? 1 2 3 4 5 6 7 8 9 10

Why do you like some areas of your body, and not others? What could you do to change the way you look? Would time help (or is time the villain)? What about better eating? Exercise? A more positive mental outlook? Perhaps a change in what may be a "misbelief" about your body? What would be your rewards if you had the kind of body you feel you'd like to have?

MIRROR, MIRROR ON THE WALL . . .

For any number of reasons, when we see ourselves in a mirror, we are almost always drawn first to what we don't like. Most people are uncomfortable in acknowledging the more positive physical attributes of their bodies. Why is this? Remember that our culture sends us loud, screaming messages—particularly to women—about how our bodies should look if we are to feel good about ourselves. (I've written about this extensively in my book, *Losing Weight Permanently: Secrets of the 2% Who Succeed,* [Shaw, 1996]). But who has the right to say how you should look? And who gives them that power? You don't have to look like Cindy Crawford or Tom Cruise to feel good about yourself. If that were the primary criterion for your self-esteem, it's conceivable you could live the rest of your life in sorrow. Comparison is always a fast track to misery.

WORK WITH THE RIGHT INFORMATION

What's the answer? God made us in such a way that we truly can influence our physical shape. However, it's usually the emotional—and unrealistic—issues that dictate how we feel we should look. We do have ways to reshape our bodies (exercise, better eating, positive mental outlook, dealing with our past, living expectantly for our future, and so forth), but it's the *emotional* issues that keep us stuck, dictating how we feel our bodies should look. So here's the formula: You must be ready emotionally—armed with up-to-date realistic information—to reshape your body physically.

I'm not saying this will be easy, but it is vital if you and I are to have bodies we can love. And since they are all we have, wouldn't it be a good idea to make our body our friend? To help us do this, let's look at some critical decisions we must make.

- Because our bodies change over time—through the natural course of aging—it is unrealistic to expect them to remain static. Flab and double chins may appear. "Spare tires" are almost inevitable. Cellulite—evil monster that it is—will continue to plague women's bodies. So here's the first decision: We must be willing to recognize that our bodies will ultimately all head south—and that our most noble efforts will not entirely reverse the process. This is called being realistic. That's the way life is, and it's an issue we'd be wise to accept and simply put to rest.

- Our bodies require consistent, tender, loving care, and ongoing maintenance. Just as we need to nurture ourselves spiritually and emotionally, we must also nurture ourselves physically—which means we need to take care of our bodies through exercise, the right kinds of vitamins, antioxidants, and high-grade food supplements. So the second decision that must be made is this: We must be committed to a consistent nurturing of our bodies as a new life pattern. It must become as natural as breathing. We will not be able to reverse the aging process, but we certainly can look—and feel—better along the way.

- This decision begins with a question: Will we commit to body care because we want to be body wise—even when we do not see immediate results? In a society that expects results in five minutes or less, this is a tough one. But it's a critical decision. You and I will never feel that our bodies are changing, or responding, fast enough. We'll always want to beat the clock, and do our best to keep Father Time and gravity at bay. So we must make yet a third decision: To honor our "temple" with utmost care, whether or not we are able to see an immediate result of our efforts.

The following are five important partial statements that, when completed, will give you your own appraisal of how you view your own body. They'll be your words, not mine, and therefore you have little choice but to believe that you've told yourself the truth. I'd like you to complete each thought.

1. My body really wants more _____.
2. I need physical healing in the following way:

   _____.

3. The three foods that make my body happy—and give me abundant energy—are

   _____.

4. I delight in the fact that my body

   _____.

5. If I love (give honor and respect to) my body daily, it will

   _____

   _____.

How did you do with these five statements? Did you provide yourself with some insights into how you see your own body? The best learning is always self-learning, and that's partially what you've been engaged in today. I want you to take seriously what you've said about yourself and work with your feelings about yourself during the remainder of these 21 days. Now, with that important information available to you, let's tackle Day 12 with its vital theme of how to stay in complete control when you find yourself in high-risk food situations—and how to stay in control *for good!*

LESSON OF THE DAY

Because God made my body his temple,
it is a body I am learning to love.

DAY 12

But What Do I Eat in a Restaurant?

Staying in Control in High-Risk Food Situations . . . for the Rest of Your Life

If there's any one question I get more than anything else it's this: What do I eat in a restaurant that will be healthy, keep me from feeling guilty, and make me feel good? Have you ever asked yourself this question? If so, you'll be glad to know that you've landed on Day 12.

First, let's start by exploding some myths about eating out. There are many, but we'll look at just four of them.

Myth #1: Most oriental food is healthy because it is low in fat and sugar. Fact: A stir-fried dish may hold as much as nine teaspoons of fat per serving. That's a lot! It's true that authentic Chinese dishes, for example, are mostly vegetables, with limited animal protein, but American-style Chinese food is usually just the opposite, with too much added fat and sugary sweet-and-sour sauces. So brush up on your Cantonese and ask your server to hold the oil, and, of course, no MSG, please.

Myth #2: Eat up those wonderful fast-food chicken and fish sandwiches because they're lower in fat than a greasy hamburger.

Fact: It's the exact opposite. Fried fish or chicken sandwiches have more fat and calories than a hamburger. If you're going to order one, at least choose grilled chicken and baked fish dishes. And hold the mayo.

Myth #3: All Italian food is healthy.

Fact: Take spaghetti. With a meatless marinara—or red clam sauce—it's one of the healthiest of the low-fat meals you can get in a restaurant. Add fresh Italian bread (sorry, no butter) and a simple salad (lemon wedges on the side, thank you), and you also have a low-fat feast. But now the large lady starts to sing, because fettuccine Alfredo (even the sound makes me put on pounds) gets 58% of its calories from fat. And it only gets worse. Many restaurant lasagnas contain more than 11 teaspoons of fat per serving. Yikes!

Myth #4: Chicken entrees are lowest in fat.

Fact: Chicken can be a tub of lard—even fatter than other dishes if it has been deep-fried, breaded, or smothered in a cream sauce. (Sorry, I know this is making you hungry.) Always tell your server how you want your chicken prepared—grilled or baked, with (okay, you win) a little sauce on the side.

Many years ago, if you wanted a truly healthful restaurant meal, you would have had to put on a cook's apron, go into his kitchen, and prepare it yourself. Not so today. In fact, most restaurants are now willing to prepare a meal that meets the "Healthy Heart" guidelines: low in fat, sodium, and cholesterol. A survey conducted by the National Restaurant Association indicated that most restaurant owners are now willing—and able—to modify their cuisine or service methods at the customer's request. So we're already better off. But nothing happens unless you make it happen. You can eat guilt-free (and stay on target during these entire 21 days—and for years to come) if your primary dining-out strategies are the same ones you're starting to use at home. Here are some strategies that my wife, LaFon, and I use when eating out.

FOUR STRATEGIES THAT WORK EVERY TIME

1. Limit or avoid fat altogether. (A great reason to avoid all buffets!) Order foods that are broiled, poached, roasted, grilled, baked, or steamed. Look for foods labeled "garden fresh," "in tomato base," or meats happily lying there smiling "in their own juices."

2. Scour the menu (which may take most of your dinner time, in some cases) for fruits, vegetables, grains, chicken, and fish. And then don't heap cheese on your vegetables or soak your grains in gravy. Don't cheat. You've made it this far, now make the commitment to an entire evening of healthy eating.

3. Here's a key point. If you're not assertive on this one, you'll probably grin and say, "Hey, I can't help it, Antonio brought it, and now I've got to eat it." Have only the foods you intend to eat brought to your table. If you're eating Italian one evening, tell signor Antonio you want only breadsticks, but not to bring the mound of garlic bread swimming in butter or the dessert tray. What you don't have in front of you, you will not eat. (One woman I know asks the server to bring a box *with* the meal. She immediately places half of her meal in the box, closes the lid, and has a wonderful lunch the following day.) Remember the

"triggers" we talked about earlier? Don't give yourself a reason to lose. Be assertive and stick with your plan.

4. Choose foods that are as close to their original form as possible, such as fresh, raw, or lightly steamed vegetables or fresh fruit—something that is more challenging in a restaurant—but you can find them. Be specially on the lookout for highly processed foods, then avoid them at all costs.

Would you agree that we're often so hungry before going out that we usually just jump in the car and salivate all the way to the restaurant? Here's how I want you to prepare yourself from this day forward. Never starve yourself before eating a large restaurant meal. *Before going out, eat a big, juicy apple.* The natural sugar will give you energy, and you won't have to eat the table napkin because you're starved when you get there.

And one more tip. This is a great one, but I think only we 21-Day people ever do it. When you're about halfway through with your restaurant meal, take a break. Push yourself back from the table. Keep drinking lots of water. Here's why. On average, it takes about twenty minutes for the brain to accept the message that you are full. So slow down. Take a break. Look around at the people. Engage in wonderful conversation. Then see whether you're as hungry as you thought you were twenty minutes before. Chances are, you'll feel full and can take the rest of your meal home. That gives you two meals from one successful dine-out! You'll also feel much better in the morning.

A DINING-OUT CHECKLIST

Because you are taking our 21-Day series seriously—and there's a good chance you'll be eating in more than one restaurant during these 21 days—I want to give you a "Dining-out checklist" to help you avoid last-minute decision making once you arrive at the restaurant. (You may want to make copies of this page.)

The Food Event Itself

- Who's going to be at your table? Are they friends or foes? Supportive, or there to distract you from your 21-Day plan? Go prepared.

  _____

  _____

- Who's cooking the food? (Restaurant, fast-food place, airline, deli, potluck)?

  _____

  _____

- What kind of meal will be served? (If you don't have this information, call ahead and find out. With airlines, *always* reserve your special meals in advance.)

  _____

  _____

Your Strategy

1. What are you prepared to do if high-fat appetizers are served?

   _____

   _____

2. How well-prepared will you be to handle your food choices during the meal? Will you have thought through what you want—even before you pick up the menu? (Hint: Sometimes it's good to not even look at it. Just tell your server what you want and how you want it prepared. That way, you're getting customized information and not guessing from what you see on the menu. What you think you see is not always what you get.)

3. How will you manage those who push food on you or say, "Hey, it's a party, eat this"?

   _____

   _____

4. The most important strategy question of all: What will be the payoffs for sticking with your 21-Day plan for better eating? When you remain disciplined, how do you think you'll feel the next morning? How will you feel if you "fall off the wagon"?

_____

_____

And to quote Miss Piggy, "Never eat more than you can lift!"

I've given you a lot to digest here (pardon the pun), but it's all so important. Review Day 12 before you go out to eat. Think of where you're going, what you'll be eating, and how you'll handle yourself when you get there. And don't forget to eat a piece of fresh fruit along the way. Your body will thank you . . . just as it will express gratitude for what you're about to learn in Day 13—*critical factors* to help set you free for the rest of your life.

LESSON OF THE DAY

When I go out to eat, I remain in full control of my new approach to eating.

DAY 13

Relationship Principles to Set You Free

Strategies to Create and Maintain Healthy Relationships That Build Openness and Trust

Over the course of our lives many of us will come across people and events that seem to make us sad, render us ineffective, cause us to be depressed, and put us in a position where we seem to have no recourse but to sing the blues—and eat! Some of the most common reasons for this malady are excessive weight gain or loss, problems at work, and problems with relationships that can lead to feelings of utter helplessness. But they are only symptoms of something more serious going on beneath the surface.

MELISSA'S PILGRIMAGE

Melissa—not her real name—discovered that even after achieving what she felt was an ideal weight (she had not yet learned that weight is almost never the real issue, not even after she lost more than 75 pounds), she still found herself filled with worry, dread, and anxiety. She just couldn't shake it. After consulting with her pastor and her physician, she was encouraged to come to see me to get help for her depression. After working with me for a couple of difficult months, she began to find relief from the demons within and little by little regained her energy and joy of living.

When I asked her what she thought had happened during our time together, she wrote me a letter summing up her thoughts. With her permission, I'm able to share with you the note I received:

Dear Dr. Jantz,

One of the first things you helped me understand was that I was a perfectionist. I was more interested in playing the game—in going after perfection rather than become involved in the progress of becoming healthy. I discovered I was trying so hard to be something I wasn't, that I was not being authentic with myself, with God, or with my family.

So I made a daily decision to try to be me. Just me. Nobody else. I began each day by praising God for *me*. I knew if I could be grateful, that I could also learn to become hopeful again. That's when I began to nurture my relationships in whole new ways. I began to go each week to a senior retirement home to help read to the elderly. I went for them, but, as it turned out, *it was those dear people who were there for me—and they were a big part of my healing.*

I quickly realized how my entire life seemed to be filled with toxic anger, fear, and guilt from my past. I was riddled with that stuff, and it was eating me alive. So I asked God to fill my heart instead of fueling my hunger for food and all its negative connotations. As I began to do this, I started practicing self-care, and before long I found myself feeling more self-confident. I began to fall in love with life rather than be in love with food. The one was setting me free; the other had kept me in bondage.

Suddenly I discovered what I can only call a passion for life. I was living a lifestyle of kindness. No longer did I live bouncing from wall to wall, bingeing, overeating, or hiding food from my family and eating it in the wee hours of the morning. My low impulse control that had plagued me with addictive behaviors was fading. I couldn't believe what was happening. Dr. Jantz, the most amazing thing for me was this. Even though my original problem was food—or so I thought—you almost never talked about food when we were together. You just kept talking about loving myself and others and going for little baby steps of progress rather than perfection. I thought it was a crazy approach at the time. But now I can say with confidence that the way you treated me saved my life.

I'll never forget all the diets I used to be on. I was the best calorie counter in my neighborhood. I knew the fat content of every box on the supermarket shelf. I had used every laxative and had purchased so many pieces of exercise equipment that my home looked like a fitness center. Trouble was, I never used any of it. I was always too depressed to bike my troubles away.

I also picked up a lot of false guilt from other people. Some would say to me, "Melissa, if you were more spiritual, and if you just loved God more, you would have more discipline and not eat so much." That hurt so much I can hardly talk about it. But I believed this false counsel and did everything I could to be a better Christian. However, that was not the issue, either. I've now learned to take what other people say with a grain of salt. You helped me understand the difference between true guilt and false guilt.

When I do something I know is wrong, I feel true remorse, ask for forgiveness, and move on. That's new for me. But it feels so good. False guilt is other people's stuff, and I'm not taking that on anymore.

You also helped me realize I had an overdeveloped sense of responsibility. It was easier for me to be concerned with the needs of others than to take care of myself. This meant that I never really looked inside long enough to see where Melissa needed help. Thank God, that's now history. I'm still working on tendencies toward codependency, but I'm now seeing progress (and not worrying about the perfection part).

But I guess, Dr. Jantz, the most important thing you taught me was to focus on the now. To live one day at a time—hour by hour, minute by minute. I now have a "present life." I can enjoy a sunrise or a sunset just for what it is. I'm learning to relax, and I feel God's healing of my body, soul, and spirit at every turn. In my relationships, I've moved from a regret of the past and fear of the future to enjoying my family and friends in the here and now.

I've called Day 13, "Relationship Principles to Set You Free," and I have taken each of these from Melissa's note to me. Let me summarize them for you.

RELATIONSHIP PRINCIPLES TO SET YOU FREE

1. *Be authentic.* Only when we are authentic human beings— honest with the person we see in the mirror—do we begin to make progress and no longer feel we need to be perfect. This is where we start to make our first exciting dash toward freedom. It's the foundation for healthy relationships.

2. *Praise God daily.* As we learn to become more grateful, we also become people of hope, knowing that our brighter future lies ahead . . . and our relationships with others improve.

3. *Nurture your friendships.* As we reach out to others, we begin to reduce our toxic anger, fear, and guilt—negative qualities that keep us in bondage.

4. *Fill your heart rather than fill your hunger.* Melissa reminds us that for her, self-care led to greater self-confidence, and that a love of life began to take the place of the love of food. As she did this, she began to develop healthier relationships with her family and friends.

5. *Live a life of balance.* A passion for all of life keeps us from falling victim to low-impulse control that leads to addictive behaviors. God has given us the great freedom not to do just anything . . . *but to do the right thing.* And one of those "right things" is to improve our relationships with those around us.

6. *Say good-bye to false guilt.* There is a great difference between real guilt and false guilt. One is a warning sign that we need to make amends; the other is something to throw by the wayside as worthless and hurtful. Unless we can sort out the difference, our relationships will continue to suffer.

7. *Eliminate codependent behavior.* Here we learn to reduce our overdeveloped sense of responsibility for others and begin to take care of ourselves. Life comes into balance. Joy returns to our hearts. When this happens, relationships become honest and nurturing.

8. *Focus on the now.* Melissa said, "I can enjoy a sunrise or a sunset just for what it is. I'm learning to relax, and I feel God's healing of my body, soul, and spirit at every turn." The same can happen to you, and it's my prayer that it already has.

Still, even with this exciting, newfound freedom, we're not home yet. Life *will* go on. The kids *will* get sick. Satan *will* throw roadblocks in our path ... and we *will* be human, with all our foibles and problems, which means we'll always find ourselves awash with temptation—which includes the temptation of certain foods that may be harmful to us—the theme you're now ready to embrace in Day 14.

LESSON OF THE DAY

*I am building a solid foundation
that is helping me to develop and
enjoy healthy relationships.*

DAY 14

Dealing with the Temptations of Foods

How to Face Temptation and Not Give In

First, the bad news. In an average year, a typical American (obviously not one of the 21-Day-ers) ingests the following:

- 135 pounds of refined sugar
- 55 pounds of fats and oils
- 300 cans of soda pop
- 20 pounds of candy
- 63 dozen donuts
- 50 pounds of cakes and cookies
- 20 gallons of ice cream
- 12 pounds of potato chips, corn chips, and pretzels

Forty-eight percent of all food consumed in the United States is "fast food" or convenience food, all of which is high in fat, salt, and sugar. And it is all so very tempting.

THOSE FOOD TRIGGERS AGAIN

There are fast-food ads on television, "golden arches" seemingly on every corner, promotions for Hollywood movies "when you buy one of this or two of these fast-food items," and the list of temptations goes on and on.

Do you remember back on Day 3 when we talked about certain environmental "triggers" to avoid if we are to "stay on the wagon" during these 21 days to better eating and beyond? We talked about the importance of avoiding certain restaurants (where visual cues are so strong that our car almost automatically turns into the driveway). We also mentioned the need to be careful when eating in the homes of some people—because, through experience, we already know what gastronomic temptations await us. And what about the assortment of triggers that can occur at church or social functions, where before we know it, fellowship has turned into donutship, and we start the long torturous road back to eating for comfort and camaraderie rather than for nourishment? Today I want to share additional ideas to help you deal with some temptations you are sure to meet. A key principle to remember is that *your actions follow your thoughts*. You become what you think about all day long. Good thinking leads to healthy eating. Here on Day 14, I want you to put your brain into high gear as you meet some of these temptations head-on.

Meet Temptation #1

The wonderful smells and the sight of an elaborately cooked meal are enough to drive us all to the table, knives and forks poised for the feast. Our bodies immediately begin to produce saliva, and, within seconds, our stomachs secrete an assortment of digestive juices. I call this the *setup*, because these triggers are ringing the chuck house bell saying, *Come and get it!*

If you're bored or angry or anxious about something, it can be even worse—especially if you're watching television and it's already your pattern to jump up during each commercial and have a little snack.

A helpful way to meet these temptations is to keep a food diary for ten days. Carry it with you at all times and make regular notations on what you eat, where you eat, when you eat, and how you feel as you eat. When you've identified your food triggers, then you're in a position to shift these triggers from a negative to a positive—but not until then.

For example, you may discover that television is a major trigger. If so, make yourself a rule that you'll never eat while the TV is on. You might eat an apple *before* your favorite show comes on so that you have food in your stomach, but then, that's it. No more food. Another great idea is to find something useful for your hands while watching TV. (No, *not* nibbling on chips; that doesn't count.) You might want to knit, write a letter, or do a crossword puzzle (you'll have time to complete one of these during the commercials alone).

Meet Temptation #2

If you are hurting your body with binge eating, then you either have, or are close to having, an eating disorder. In a typical binge, very high-calorie foods—such as ice cream, donuts, and other sugar-filled, high-cholesterol pastries—are eaten rapid-fire, almost as if there were no tomorrow. Unfortunately, the only thing that stops the typical binge is pain, the need to vomit, sleepiness, or an interruption. Here are some ways to help you meet this temptation:

- Make a conscious effort to keep "binge" foods out of the house.
- Avoid the kinds of strict diets that will set you up for severe hunger pangs.

- Look at past binge experiences. Why did they take place? What was bothering you at the time (triggers, again)? What did you eat? Where did you get the food? Did you binge at home?

Note: If you are a binger, you *can* be helped. And I'd encourage you to see a counselor if you feel your problem is getting out of hand. But whether you get help or not, you need to develop a strategy for the future.

- Wait at least 15 minutes before you give in to the next binge. Take that quarter of an hour to do something else: Take a walk, talk with a friend, read a psalm. During that time, you distract yourself enough, hopefully, so that the binge never takes place.
- If you feel a binge coming on, drink a tall glass of water or eat an apple or some other high-fiber food. You want the fullness in your stomach to stave off your urge to binge.

No question about it, bingeing is a serious health problem. That's why it's important that you consider getting help in developing a weight-management program that encourages gradual weight loss by doing everything we're learning during our 21 days together. If bingeing is a problem for you, I want you to know that I understand, and I'm praying for your full recovery.

Meet Temptation #3

The water issue. Your temptation will be not to drink enough—and to feel that you don't need it because you don't feel thirsty. That's when you may need it most. When tempted to overeat, binge, gorge, or respond to your environmental triggers, drink water. Our bodies' demand for water is second only to the demand for air, and yet we never drink enough. None of us do.

So, drink more water. It's the cheapest, best, most digestive-efficient liquid you can put into your body. Buy a sports bottle and keep it filled with water at all times. Keep one in your car, in the kitchen, next to your computer, on your desk at the office. Drink when you're thirsty and drink when you're not. I keep a full liter bottle on my desk at all times, and I don't leave the office until I've finished it—sometimes two or more. Be known as a drinker—*of water*.

OPTIMUM HEALTH ... FOR PENNIES A DAY

Water helps metabolize fat, helps organs function, brings healing to sore muscles and joints, and prevents dehydration—and those are only a few of the benefits of water. It's the best way to meet almost any food temptation. Here's a thought to highlight: *Most of the time you and I are not hungry. We are just bored, or anxious, or don't know what to do with ourselves.* So rather than open the fridge and start grazing, drink water. Do this for five straight days and see what happens (make an entry in your food diary as to how you feel). Yes, you may need to urinate more regularly, but your bladder will quickly adjust after a few weeks, and you'll be just fine. Have I been on my "water soapbox" long enough? I hope I've persuaded you to give your body what it wants most: water. It's one of the best, most effective ways to deal with the temptation of foods—and it will cost you only pennies a day, a meager price for producing a healthier, happier body—one that you can truly come to love and appreciate.

This final note on Day 14. If we don't confront our food temptations, we will set ourselves up for even more stress, anxiety, and guilt. The more stress we place on our minds and bodies, the greater desire we'll have to eat, and the more difficult it will be to handle the temptations that will surely come our way. So let's take another, closer look at a plan that deals with this stress: one of the chief villains that keeps us from developing better eating habits—the subject of Day 15.

LESSON OF THE DAY

I am confronting my food temptations by being prepared to meet my challenges head-on, knowing I can be successful.

DAY 15

Develop an Action Plan for Stress

Having a Weight Challenge Does Not Necessarily Result from a Lack of Willpower; It's Often a Response to Stress

We want to eat for two primary reasons: to feel better and improve our mood or to raise our energy level. In one way or the other, the food we eat is both a mood- and energy-altering substance that helps create a balance between our body and our mind. What happens to many of us, however, is that we eat more for mood than for food, and mood is more closely tied to stress—that ill-advised, ill-timed compensation for not taking care of ourselves emotionally. When we eat out of stress, we set ourselves up for a compulsive, toxic buildup that often leads to bingeing and weight gain.

Here are five typical food "stressors" and solutions on how to deal with them.

FOOD STRESS #1:

The problem: You eat the same food over and over, misbelieving that there are only a few "safe foods." This misguided thinking may have come from your background where you were told that some foods were good and some bad. (I'll confess right here that large portions of broccoli are still a challenge for me—and after all these years!)

The solution: Go for variety. For example, they don't have to be *boring veggies*. Try fresh fruits, whole grains, fiber, different kinds of pastas. Some, admittedly, may not be your favorite at the outset, but when you begin to appreciate their nutrient value—because you're committed to better eating—you'll discover they are not so bad at all. Before long, your car will zoom right by those fast-food franchises. It won't happen overnight. Remember the premise of this book: *It takes 21 days to form a new habit or way of eating.*

FOOD STRESS #2:

The problem: Retaining old mental "labels" perpetuates food stress.

The solution: Relabel or rename foods that you've previously considered unsafe. For example, you may regard certain foods as "evil" or "binge" foods or "unsafe" foods. But food is food. It's what you "feel" about foods that taint them. Some people binge on nuts. Nothing wrong with nuts. Some binge on fruit. There's nothing wrong with fruit. There *is* something wrong when a person binges on nuts and fruit, but it's not the nuts and the fruit that's the problem. It's a person's *use* of the food as a vehicle for inappropriate behavior that's the problem. If you have considered certain "foods" as unsafe, then reconsider. Unless the food is blatantly high-fat, loaded with sodium, and has more cholesterol than should be allowed by law, it's not as much the food as it is *the attitude toward the food.*

That's why maintaining old mental food labels creates such tremendous stress. Again, you have options. Exercise them.

Think beyond the old labels. Move past what you've been thinking about certain foods until now.

FOOD STRESS #3:

The problem: We feel we cannot celebrate or acknowledge special days with food. This is a huge issue for many who are trying to manage their weight. They often misbelieve that cake, pie, and ice cream are out of their lives forever. Life is no more fun, and they figure they'll just have to grin and bear it. If you believe this, you're setting yourself up for unbelievable stress.

The solution: Celebrate special days with appropriate "acknowledgment foods." If it's your anniversary or your birthday or a baptism or you're celebrating a child's christening, enjoy yourself, have a party, invite your friends, and have a piece (one piece!) of cake and some ice cream (one scoop). That's the wonderful stuff that parties are made of. If you don't get into the mood of your celebration, you may start feeling stressed immediately. Note this: Most people I see who try not to eat cake and ice cream on special occasions usually binge later in private. If this is you, just know you don't have to do this anymore. (Just invite me to the party, and we'll talk about it . . . over *one piece* of cake!)

FOOD STRESS #4:

The problem: Playing the game of "clean plate" wars leads to an inordinate amount of food stress. Perhaps this is how you were raised: *Remember the starving children in China. Clean your plate.* As a child, I always wondered if my parents actually sent my leftovers to Beijing. I don't think they did, but they somehow felt that the ploy would work to get me to eat all that was placed before me. The problem of feeling that we need to clean our plate at all costs can continue, however, well beyond childhood.

The solution: Readjust your portions. Having a "portion plan" keeps you from stressing out. Try this tonight at dinner, and you'll feel better immediately. If the portions on your plate are too large—or seem so—and you are still a charter member of the "clean plate club," you will overeat. Bingo. Stress. So your solution is simple: Put less on your plate—yes, even in restaurants you can ask for smaller portions—and you will avoid the "full plate" syndrome (the "I-ordered-it, now I've-got-to-eat-it-problem") that invariably translates to an over-full stomach. Just ask for smaller portions.

FOOD STRESS #5:

The problem: Pushy people can set you up for food stress. These are folks who try to persuade you to feel guilty because you don't eat enough ("My, you eat just like a little bird ... come on, fill up that plate now"). Or if you're at a buffet (something I highly discourage), they'll say, "Aren't these plates small? We'll just have to go back for seconds. Come on, join me." And it's back to the feeding trough for more of the stuff that nobody needs. These people have not yet learned to hear the words *No, thanks.* Undealt with, this will cause you an enormous amount of food stress.

The solution: Just say no. Prepare for the food event in advance (as we discussed in Day 12 when we created a "Dining-out checklist"). Have some nutritious high-fiber food before you go out with these people (there's our trusty juicy apple again) and you'll find it a lot easier to deal with the food pushers in your life. Make the decision now not to buy into their agenda—whatever it might be. You don't need to be mean or try to make them feel guilty. Just take care of yourself. Both your body and your raised spirits will thank you.

Keep in mind that you may not be successful with any one of the above solutions immediately. That's why it's important that you keep working on them for the full 21 days and beyond. We'll never be able to avoid the source of food stressors completely, but we *can* diminish their effects. You are too important not to take the mild risks to make it happen.

POSITIVE STRESS CREATES POSITIVE CHANGE

A final note: Creating healthy eating habits during these 21 days can be stressful in itself. *But positive stress also creates positive change* (and sometimes it can be painfully positive), out of which comes joy, peace, and a lifestyle that starts to make sense—finally.

How did you do with today's subject? I hope it didn't stress you out too much. But if it did, I'm assuming it was a positive form of stress, which, I promise you, will produce some exciting, positive change in your life within the next few days . . . as long as you give it a try and then stay with it.

Now we're going to turn to another critical issue—something that's not often written about. It's how to deal with better eating and its relationship to potential biological time bombs. This means a spirited discussion of the many things we can do to improve our immune systems. So if you're ready to keep going, let's move on to Day 16 and defuse the bomb.

LESSON OF THE DAY

My weight challenge is not necessarily because of my lack of willpower but rather, my natural reaction to stress.

DAY 16

Defuse Biological Time Bombs

Bringing Health to Your Immune System

What would you give if you could live effectively with virtually all the cycles of life? This would mean you'd be levelheaded, not prone to fits of frustration, enjoy a strong immune system, and maintain an ideal weight at all times. Now, you might say, if we could put *that* into a pill we'd all be living on Easy Street.

I'm not going to promise you the world here on Day 16, but I think we can get a little closer to dealing with some of the crucial issues that often keep us off balance, out of sorts, and out of shape.

First of all, cycles are what life is all about. There is a cycle to the seasons, the cycles of age—from young to old, cycles of trends in clothing, music, art, and other forms of entertainment. Our very existence is built around cycles. The purpose of life cannot realistically be to alter these cycles but to live in harmony with them and make them work for us. And that's the challenge.

Have you checked out the anti-aging advertisements lately? I don't know about your newspaper, but I'm seeing more of these ads every day in mine. Each seems to be ballyhooing the next fountain of youth: a cream to reduce unwanted wrinkles and a pill to give you back a figure and a face you haven't seen in your mirror for years. This may all seem harmless enough, but I need to provide a warning: *Beware of buying into an anti-aging orientation.* Yes, you can do a few things to reshape how you look. But realistically, the clock will continue to tick, and you and I will naturally "cycle" ourselves into the next phase of our lives. So rather than think anti-aging, let's think *vibrant living.* That's what you and I really want, isn't it?

Vibrant living is a choice. An attitude. Yes, certain numbers of us may have serious health issues to deal with sooner or later. I understand that. Some will get cancer, arthritis, or other debilitating diseases. But there is one issue—obesity—that does not fall into the category of "I can't help it . . . I just got it!" Obesity is the number one most preventable cause of death, because *it's all about choices.* No one really chooses to get cancer or diabetes. Yet, every day, people choose to become obese by their lifestyle and their lack of attention to the foods they put in their mouths.

KEY FACTS OF BETTER EATING AND HUMAN BIOLOGY

If you are feeling lethargic, out of condition, and out of sorts—and this has been going on for some time—I would certainly recommend that you consult your physician. But for most of us, our condition can simply be traced to how we eat. Here's the good news. A change to better eating at any point in our life will result in numerous benefits such as more energy, better digestion, improved blood pressure, and a more effective metabolism, to mention only a few.

Even with the advent of health concerns or disease, our food choices will make a tremendous difference, because through better eating we can strengthen the functioning of our immune systems and maintain a healthy weight. God's Word tells us we are "fearfully and wonderfully made" (Ps. 139:14). This means the machine called the body was designed to operate at peak performance. The question always is *what kind of fuel are we putting in the tank?*

WHAT'S GOING INTO THE TANK?

If, for example, there's not enough fiber in our diet, the other substances in our intestines will just sit there, fermenting and stagnating. Any toxic material from food or substances created by bacteria would have just that much more time to be in contact with our intestinal walls. So what we eat *does* matter. Fiber is but one example. Similar unhappy things happen inside us when we take in too much LDL (low density lipoprotein) cholesterol (the bad kind), allowing it to carry cholesterol to our arteries where it will create plaque and set us up for a possible heart condition. We become what we eat, so let's continue to guard against putting faulty fuels into our tank.

CHANGING YOUR METABOLISM

And then there's metabolism—the physical and chemical process in an organism by which protoplasm is produced, maintained, and destroyed, and by which energy is made available. The metabolic process, for most of us, can be improved by better food habits and exercise. Even in those rare disorders such as hypothyroidism, a person can feel better when better food choices are made.

I've seen many people lose weight—and keep it off—even though they had stubborn metabolic issues going against them. Is it a challenge? Yes. Is it possible for better eating to make a difference in how we feel as we grow older? Absolutely! Good food choices can move us toward a greater sense of well-being. That's how God made us.

WHAT ABOUT SPECIAL SITUATIONS?

I wonder how many millions of anti-gas pills and antacid tablets and potions are sold in the country in a given year. It's incredible how many people will unthinkingly keep eating poorly, put lousy "gas" into their tank, then take a couple "cure-all" tablets and expect their problem to go away. It won't. The pill is just another mask that prevents the ailment from presenting itself.

Some folks imagine that a condition such as heartburn is a biological (age) factor. In most cases, it's not. If we have overeaten—binged—during the earlier part of our life, the stomach's digestion will be seriously affected, making us overproduce inordinate amounts of acid. The body is a smart machine: The more acid it feels it needs, the more it will produce. Just as in economics, the stomach, too, knows all about supply and demand. The hyperacid condition is what creates the after-meal burning. The acid comes in contact with our esophagus, and voilà! Heartburn.

A caution: *Be careful about overusing antacids.* A more effective means of control is to try walking for fifteen minutes and drinking water. When you do this, you're dealing with the real issues of health and not masking them with over-the-counter remedies. I know too many people who eat everything but the tablecloth—followed by a rich dessert—with the idea of eating antacids after dinner. This is the nonthinking person's way to weight gain, poor health, and obesity. The real key, of course, is to eat less and make better food choices (i.e., consuming less fat, less bad cholesterol, more fiber, less salt, less sugar, more raw fruits, and so forth). It will take the body some time to adapt to this new, high-octane fuel, but remember: It took us a while to get into our present condition. It is unrealistic to expect changes overnight. Before long, however, the pings and knocks in our body's engine will be things of the past. If you are not eating properly now, it will probably take a full 21 days for you to get into the habit, but when you finally do, you will have a standard of excellence to measure your progress against for the rest of your life. The good news is that we really can avoid the biological and health time bombs by learning to eat better now ... doing it one day at a time.

MENOPAUSE AND CRAVINGS

There are chemical changes going on in our bodies all the time, and they are especially upsetting during menopause. Again, how women care for themselves does affect how their bodies respond to their God-planned body clocks—clocks he designed.

Among the more common complaints among women during menopause are the cravings that often lead to bingeing and overeating, which lead to consistently poor food choices, which lead to weight gain, which lead to feeling bad about themselves for the "terrible" things they've done to their body. Here's some good news about cravings (actually good news for *everyone*— men and women, menopausal or not):

1. They don't last forever.
2. Drinking a liter of water during a craving will help you avoid overeating or bingeing, 80% of the time.
3. Instead of running off to eat the food you crave, make yourself wait 15 minutes. This allows you enough time to renew your strength and remember your goals; and in most instances, the craving will pass.

Better eating habits will give you more energy and provide you with heightened self-confidence. Greater self-confidence means better decisions. Do you see the pattern here—the pattern of living vibrantly at any age? It *can* be accomplished. You do *not* have to wait until your biological time bomb explodes. You can bring in the nutrition bomb squad now. In fact, you brought in the team when you made your commitment of 21 days to better eating.

Since I'm already Johnny-one-note on this, I'll say it again: *You're after progress, not perfection.* Just keep on doing what you are doing now in this program. Success is your daily pursuit of a worthwhile goal . . . and the fact that you've pursued your goals and kept your commitments through Day 16 tells me that you are on the road to great success. This reminder is all the more important as we move into Day 17, where we now bring in another powerhouse team to help provide damage control in the event you fall off the wagon.

LESSON OF THE DAY

I don't have to wait for the biological time bomb to explode. I can defuse it through better eating and weight management.

Damage Control for Binges

Bringing Your Life Back into Focus

Gloria was a binger. No one knew it. Not her husband, her children, or her friends. On the surface, it seemed as if Gloria had it all together. She was active in church and the PTA, took her kids to soccer and music lessons, and easily could have been voted the best all-around-mom in her community.

But her nasty little secret was slowly killing her. She felt lonely, sad, and terrible about herself—all the time. She had binged for so long that to "come clean" would have been a huge embarrassment. So, without getting help, things just got worse. Her obsessive-compulsive behavior caused her to squirrel away food, eat it quickly—and in great amounts—vomit, and then eat more. It was the worst thing that had ever happened to Gloria in her life. Only when she felt she'd come to the end of her rope did she come to me for help.

Binges. However defined, binges are a food behavior that's symptomatic of how bad one feels about him- or herself. Binges make us feel out of control and that there's something wrong with us. And they're always done in secret. In all the binge cases I've counseled, prior to an actual binge there has usually been a great deal of disappointment, frustration, anger, fear, or guilt. All unresolved and undealt with. Wrongly, those who binge feel they have found a creative way to cope with their problems—a coping mechanism that seems to bring comfort and numb the pain.

Bingeing is *not* the answer. And if you fall into this category of unhealthy behavior, I have good news for you. You can be helped . . . and you can be cured. Let's look at some primary steps to help in binge control:

- *Realize that there is a learning curve to controlling binges.* No one ever stops bingeing instantly. You may have been on autopilot so long that you have lost all objectivity when it comes to a possible solution for your eating disorder. A primary key to binge control is to know your food triggers (Day 14). Again, take out your food diary and see what's been going on. Often, you will be your most effective teacher—if you listen to your own wisdom. What is your pattern? Where do you binge? Why? What is the prelude to your bingeing? Knowing your *emotional* triggers will take longer to identify and figure out. But as you work on understanding the whys, hows, and whens of bingeing, your knowledge will at least keep you running toward your goal. And if you drop the ball, it's okay. Just pick it up again and keep moving toward your objective. You can be free from your bondage, and you can know that freedom today.
- *Forgive yourself—daily.* Learning forgiveness is one of the primary means for recovery from bingeing. Just going through the motions won't cut it. It's critical that you squarely face your feelings of fear, hurt, and inadequacy

and learn to say to the person in the mirror, *I forgive you.* Forgiving yourself is not the same as excusing yourself. Forgiving yourself allows for the learning curve to play its complete role. If you don't say, "Self, I'm sorry; I forgive me," then you will store all manner of resentments against yourself and the blame game begins once again. Instead, tell yourself, "Today is a new day for me. Today I get to practice making new choices. I am doing this with God's help. I am comfortable taking today's baby steps on my way to food freedom."

- *Forgive others—daily.* The Bible reminds us to not let the sun go down on our anger. If you go to bed at night filled with angry, toxic feelings, you will tend to continue to blame others for your problems and anxieties, and you may never learn to take full responsibility for your own actions. For the serious overeater, an unforgiving spirit is a prelude to bingeing. If this is your challenge, perhaps this verse from Psalm 51:10 could be your motto: "Create in me a clean heart, O God, and renew a right spirit within me" (KJV). Here's the pattern: unforgiveness → resentments →toxic emotional state → release of frustrations through bingeing → guilt → shame. Anger and frustration with friends and family—left unresolved—will send you tumbling down the staircase to defeat faster than anything else I can think of. But it doesn't have to be that way for you ever again.
- *Remove "setup" foods.* These are the foods you normally use to binge on. Get rid of them. Don't buy them anymore. Don't even go down that aisle in the supermarket. Don't squirrel them away in a cupboard or the spare bedroom. Even as you progress in controlling your bingeing, don't become overconfident. Remove the "setup" foods from your living environment. Period! You also need to be aware that you may be doing a "mental" setup for a binge—something that can happen slowly and subtly. You know your own

pattern, because you'll be able to read about it in your food diary. If you find you're doing a mental "setup," you'll need to stop and evaluate what's recently been going on to bring you to this point. Review the above three steps often, and then recheck all the ways you may be setting yourself up. Then reenergize your living environment to fortify the "silent energy" of the setup—that unspoken environment that has been your own private playground for bingeing. Play different kinds of music (many bingers actually create an unholy ritual when bingeing). Try wearing different clothes. Rearrange your cabinets, closets, or wherever the lethal material (binge food) is stored.

- *Refocus and regroup.* When you're about to binge, immediately begin *renewing your mind and spirit with God.* He is the source of your healing. He created your body to eat healthy foods and to eat them in a healthy manner. Pray when you feel the hurt and shame coming on. Let God know how you feel, how you want to be different, and ask him to bless your present and future efforts. And then thank him, in advance, for giving you the courage to say no. Not going to God at once can create a gap in your recovery. Seeking him immediately helps you refocus on your goal of *eating better and safely* more quickly and allows you to reenergize yourself before other distractions creep in and push you off the edge once more. And while you seek the Father's face, be sure you continue to drink water, go for brisk walks—doing your part to bring you back to what you know is healthful living.

- *Read aloud one or more of the many affirmations we've already presented in this book.* Reaffirm who you are, the objectives you want to accomplish, and why it's important that you accomplish them. Here is one more affirmation to help you along the way:

I forgive myself at all times. I know I'm not where I want to be, but I also know I'm not where I once was. I thank you, God, for the courage and strength you're pouring into my life, and I am eternally grateful. I see myself as whole, well, and eating better each day. Thank you for loving me enough to make me the person you designed me to be.

Eleanor Roosevelt once said, "Friendship with oneself is all-important, because without it one cannot be friends with anyone else in the world." You were not meant to be an island of hurt surrounded by a sea of despair. We all have physical, spiritual, and emotional challenges—although they may not be of the same form or making. That's why we need each other—so we can be vulnerable to one another and in that vulnerability find peace and rest. This fact alone will speed you toward recovery, and with God's help you will be known as one who has a heart of hope—the uplifting, encouraging theme of Day 18.

LESSON OF THE DAY

I'm not yet where I want to be, and I'm not what I'm going to be, but thank God I'm not what I used to be. I'm making measurable progress in reasonable time.

Nurture a Heart of Hope

Grateful People Nourish Themselves with God and Others

I want to ask you a couple of questions as we come closer to the end of our 21 days together. They're simple but important. First: Which part of an egg is most important? The shell, the albumen, or the yoke? Or second: Which member of a family is most important: the mother, father, or the children? Difficult to answer, you say. Take the egg. Without the shell, there's no protection; without the albumen we wouldn't be able to enjoy an egg without eating its cholesterol; and without the yoke there could be no chickens to provide us with future eggs.

And what about a family? Without a father, there would be no sperm; with no mother there would be no eggs; and without the children there would be no one to call mother and father. Here's where I'm going with this: You and I are wonderfully and intricately made. We have a body, soul, and spirit. Within our body we have organs, bones, blood, flesh, and a vast network of tiny, complicated nerves that keep us active, in motion, vibrant, and alive. What's more important? A bone or a nerve? A sinew or an artery? Impossible questions to answer.

YOU ARE ONE WHOLE PERSON

We cannot isolate one part of our body and say it's more important than another any more than we can say one part of an egg, or a valued member of our family, is more important than others. That's why what you are reading in *21 Days to Better Eating* is a whole person—wholistic—approach. What we *think* affects how we eat. The issues we allow to remain unresolved affect how we think about food: Our emotions are inextricably tied to our behavior. It's all one piece. And that's why in Day 18 you'll see how a heart of hope—something that, on the surface, may not seem to have much at all to do with eating well, or taking care of our physical bodies—plays an enormous role. A *heart of hope* is a heart of gratitude rather than resentment, for resentment is one of the primary reasons for overeating, bingeing, and the avoidance of self-care. A heart of hope knows that a loving God is our ultimate healer. A heart of hope knows how vital it is to love, accept, and forgive—three of its most important attributes.

ALL OF YOU IS IMPORTANT

When we overload our bodies with food as a means of comforting ourselves, using food to attempt to deal with unresolved pain, anger, or frustration, we leave no room for the spirit to live and breathe. Instead of opening our hearts to others, we are more prone to tune out, isolate ourselves, watch television endlessly, go about listlessly, or sleep off the effects of a binge.

This is not the kind of normal activity God intended for you and me. He wants us to have hearts of hope for today and tomorrow. When this is our objective, we will want to keep food in its proper perspective, eating no more than what's necessary to keep our minds keen and our bodies in a proper state of alertness and readiness for action. Do you see the analogy to the egg and to the family? Every component of your life is important. No part is more important than another.

So with the many challenges you are facing today, how do you develop and maintain your heart of hope? How do you fix in your mind that without hope, it will be terribly difficult to manage other areas of your life? Let's look at two of the most loving things you can do to help create your heart of hope. First, learn to be a friend. Friends share the same feelings of vulnerability. They listen to each other. They suffer together, laugh together, play together, and enjoy life together. They also share many of the same risks, because "playing it on the edge" creates a bond, just as mountain climbers—roped together—consider themselves as one unit, linked together, often from a bond of mutual support as much as anything.

GIVE AWAY YOUR SMILE

Being a friend also means to be transparent. This is often the tough part ... *If my friend only knew who I really am, she would not like me; she might even reject me, and I just can't handle that possibility.* Yes, that is a risk, but I think you'll find it's more of a risk in your mind than in reality. If you are to create a heart of hope, then you must take those "baby step" risks to become the whole, integrated person of hope your Creator designed you to be.

Are you willing to stretch yourself a little in the days ahead in the friendship department? You may start by just smiling more at the waitress in the restaurant; saying thank-you to the young person who bags your groceries at the supermarket; by telling your spouse and your children how special they are and how fortunate you are to be part of their lives. In doing these "little" things that are, in fact, not little at all, you are building the foundation for your heart of hope. And here is an attitude that will literally win the day for you: *Give your love and friendship freely, expecting nothing in return.* Do this and your heart will grow big and strong, and you'll discover there's more love there than you ever imagined.

SHOES ON THE TRACKS

As the great Indian leader Mahatma Gandhi stepped aboard a train one day, one of his shoes slipped from his foot and landed on the track beneath him. The train had already begun to move, so he wasn't able to retrieve his lost shoe. To the bewilderment of his friends who saw this incident, Gandhi quietly took off the other shoe and threw it back along the track so that it would land close to the first. Asked why he'd done such a thing, Gandhi smiled back, "The poor man who finds the shoe lying on the track," he said, "will now have a pair he can use." Gandhi possessed a heart of hope and love and compassion and an abiding concern for others.

I love this story because it's a reminder of how you and I could be living our lives if we choose to: always one step ahead of anxiety, so "love alert" that common worries and frustrations no longer derail us but instead give us even greater reasons to be creative in our love.

Do you have a "shoe"—and a smile—to give away today to someone who doesn't have any to wear? Perhaps it's a colleague at work, your spouse, your children, a friend you haven't talked to for many years. When you give yourself to others, your heart of hope and joy will not be far behind.

ALWAYS TELL THE TRUTH

Another major ingredient to help you create a heart of hope is to tell the truth. Always. Live your life so that the truth will always be known as your friend. Just as you want to enjoy food freedom—to be free to eat the right things for the right reasons at the right time—so must you also seek the exciting freedom that truth can provide for every area of your life. Have you noticed that we always have to explain ourselves when we lie (and we'd also better have a great memory!)? This is the crazy material that TV sitcoms are made of: funny on television, not so cute in real life. But *truth* is its own explanation. It's your guaranteed cure for confusion. You may have tried to make food your comfort up until now, but it hasn't worked. However, when you are loyal to the truth and make it your central focus, it can be your comfort for a lifetime.

If a heart of hope is anything, it is truth. The more truth, the less stress; the more truth, the less anxiety; the more truth, the greater and stronger your courage; the more truth, the less codependency; the more truth, the fewer sleepless nights. Tell the truth, and your healing begins. Live the truth, and your life will never again be the same.

I realize that Day 18 has been a different kind of day—more reflective, perhaps, than other days. I also sincerely pray that you'll put what you've learned here into practice immediately. To help you do this, here are some suggestions to help you begin to cultivate the art of friendship and speaking the truth today and throughout the *many* 21 days of your life that lie ahead.

- To be a friend today, I'm prepared to

  _____

- In my commitment to tell the truth, I'm going to start by

  _____

- I will know I'm creating a heart of hope when I

_____

_____

Well, we have only three days to go. Congratulations on hanging in there and for keeping your 21-day commitment to learning how to live better and feel better through better eating habits. Earlier in the book, we talked about the importance of maintaining healthy emotional boundaries and their strong relationship to how we view food. Now, as we move to Day 19, we're going to get more specific with one of those boundaries as we work through one of the most complex issues of all, something I call the "Dance of Sex and Weight."

LESSON OF THE DAY

*Friendship and truth are two of my goals as
I seek to create a heart of hope.*

The Dance of Sex and Weight

"Sexy" Sells. But Does It Really Deliver?

The headline on the cover of the magazine screamed: *Take off five pounds fast! Melt away your Thanksgiving binge.* Inside was a full-color piece titled "Celebrity Inspiration . . . How the stars drop five pounds fast." For Shelley Fabares, it's a "magic drink" that keeps her at her ideal weight of 118 pounds. Candice Bergen turns to her "Paris plan," a bowl of onion soup for lunch and dinner and a banana or apple for breakfast. Dolly Parton likes to "juice it up" by enjoying squeezed orange juice for breakfast, papaya juice for lunch, and a glass of apple cider for dinner for up to five days to stay at her trim 105 pounds. A subhead tells us that Whitney Houston likes to "binge on eggs," and when Sharon Stone wants to lose a quick five, she sits down to a sumptuous meal of celery and carrots.

RED-FLAG ALERT

These are the quick-fix, lose-five-pounds-fast regimens of just a few of the twelve ravishing women featured in the article, and at first glance their methods of attacking fat may seem to be just the ticket for optimum weight management. Who wouldn't want a surefire way to lose a fast five pounds? It all seems so right, so okay, so all-American. So *everybody's doing it.* However, what should alarm us is one of the captions over the full-color pictures of ever-so-thin Dolly Parton, Joan Collins, Cybill Shepherd, and Sharon Stone that read,

"Lose that holiday weight and look great with diet strategies from the experts: stars who have to look slim for parties, parts, and public appearances."

I hope you will not buy into this fraudulent claim. Marketing their images by appearing voluptuous, trim, and sexy, and latching on to various diets to guarantee their thinness has always been important for the celebrity women who grace the pages of the magazine. But for the article to attempt to tie YOU to their overnight strategies so that YOU, too, will look good during the holidays—or on any other day of the year—is deceptive. It is an attempt to span an almost unbridgeable gap.

If you do happen to achieve overnight success with one of these plans, the diet could hook you inappropriately and catapult you into yet another backwash of dieting gimmicks. If it doesn't work—and the article makes no promise it will—then it's just one more fad that you've tried and failed.

The piece says nothing about looking "healthy" for the holidays but focuses only on the quickest way to lose five pounds. Is this article going to ruin your life? I don't think so. However, if you read articles like this over and over, week after week, year after year, and try every diet by "experts" that suggests immediate success so that you, too, can achieve and maintain your own personal celebrity look, then, yes, it will do you harm—especially if you are already challenged with obsessive-compulsive food behaviors.

DONNA'S STORY

In her own words, here's what nineteen-year-old Donna (not her real name) told me in a private session. I share these thoughts with you with her permission.

Every time I went to the supermarket I would buy a copy of the latest tabloid and at least two or three glamour and fitness magazines. I would carefully cut out those beautiful bodies, copy their diets, and post them on my refrigerator. Then I'd tackle their suggestions one by one: I'd juice for a few days, then I'd starve myself for a while, then I would drink tea for a week, then I'd exercise nonstop to the point of physical and mental exhaustion. What drove me to keep trying to lose weight was all these beautiful, big-busted, attractive Hollywood models I'd taped to my refrigerator door. I'd made them my idols. But nothing ever worked. I'd lose a couple pounds, look in the mirror, and still not be satisfied with the shape of my body, get disgusted with myself, and then go on a binge by opening the refrigerator (refusing to look at the celebrities staring at me from the door), and clean out whatever was inside. Then I'd feel guilty, promising myself I would never diet and never worship all those movie and television stars or binge again, only to find myself two days later back at the same supermarket checkout stand, picking up yet another sensational tabloid and secretly praying this time, "Please, God, make it work. If they can be beautiful, thin, and sexy, so can I."

THE JOY OF SEX VERSUS
THE JOY OF COOKING

Donna does what millions do—and it's not just women: They equate how they look (thoughts that come from how, what, and how often they eat) to how they feel about themselves sexually. There's no question that eating and sexuality are closely connected. People say they are "hungry for sex" and "hungry for food." We see books such as *The Joy of Sex* and *The Joy of Cooking*. We use our thoughts, senses, and fantasies both for oral and sexual appetites.

We're not going to change this. Nor should we try. This is how we have been wired. The key is to understand the similarities of the two appetites and not allow one to be so powerful that it over-influences the other.

Since you have been faithful with our program to better eating habits, I'm sure that you're beginning to see some significant changes in your life. This is because you've shifted your thinking from *weight* to *health*. You've started to see food in an entirely different light, you look healthier, and have perhaps lost a few pounds. Now take a look in the mirror. The person staring back at you is starting to look very good. At this point, it's important that you ask yourself a couple of questions about some of the sexual challenges you may now—or may soon—be facing. I know you'll be honest in your answers . . .

1. As I eat better and look better, I may receive more sexual attention from others. How am I supposed to deal with an appreciative opposite sex? Can my overall goals of well-being remain greater than my most immediate fears—particularly of the opposite sex paying more attention to me? If it is your objective to be a person who's committed to physical, spiritual, and emotional growth—the core of our 21-day program—for the rest of your life, this could

indeed be an issue for you. But it is a risk you must take if you're to come to grips with the real issue at stake: to achieve a healthy balance in every area of your life. You will find comfort in seeking counsel from your two "accountability" friends or group. And remember to ask God to guide and lead you as you move into what may be uncharted waters.

2. Will I be able to trust myself? If I begin to look better, lose a few pounds, start to feel my sexuality—and actually learn to accept the attention I receive from the opposite sex—will I compromise my values? There is no need to compromise your values if you remain committed to your goal of better living through better eating. This will, however, be one of those "high dive" experiences that you may have to experience to fully understand. You will learn a lot about yourself as you stay on this program—not just for 21 days but for the rest of your life. It may be frightening at first. But just because you begin looking better, your values don't need to change. Until now, you may have been hiding your God-given sexuality behind a wall of fat. Now you have the exciting privilege of being—and expressing—the whole person you've always been.

WHAT HEALTHY PEOPLE DO

People like you who succeed in looking and feeling better, because you're learning to eat better, know the concept is simple but not necessarily easy. That's why you've made the lifelong commitment to better eating. You also seek and listen to counseling that focuses on the whole person. You throw away the diet books. You stop counting calories. You learn to read the labels in the supermarket. You don't watch diet ads on television. Instead of nibbling endlessly on calorie-laden, high-fat snack foods, you eat carrots, sticks of celery, raisins, fruit, and other nutritious foods. Why? Because you have learned to like your body, and you *no longer maintain the strong, inappropriate association between food and sexuality.* You no longer dance the dance of sex and weight.

YOUR IMPROVED "SELF-TALK"

As you continue to affirm the words *I care about myself . . . I am becoming the person I was meant to be . . . I like what God has created . . . I am a person who looks good and feels good, and I don't need to compare myself with movie stars or anyone else . . .* then a new world of self-acceptance begins to unfold, carrying you yet another step closer to your goal of feeling better physically, mentally, and spiritually.

Think good thoughts of yourself. Never put yourself down. Believe in yourself—even when you don't feel you can. What you think, you are. Your subconscious hears all and believes all, so feed it positive, constructive thoughts about yourself. Treat *you* with respect.

The more you can say these words to yourself, the more you will be able to see food for what it really is—fuel for nourishment and growth. That's when you'll be able to face the pantry, the supermarket shelves, and the inside of your refrigerator and be confident that you can—and will—*win with food.* That's the subject of our next to last day together and the energizing theme of Day 20.

LESSON OF THE DAY

"Sexy" sells . . . but it never delivers.

How to Win with Food

Your Path to Permanent Weight Loss

Now that we've covered the waterfront on the subject of eating better—helping you deal with everything from the influence of mood on food, taking control of your environment, how to prevent relapses to making exercise fun again, and creating a heart of hope— now let's talk about specific combinations of food to help you continue your journey toward better eating.

What follows is *not* a diet—it's healthy eating.

It's not a rigid discipline—but rather, an exciting, sensible, healthy approach that says, Body . . . I'm going to take good care of you for the rest of my life. I'm no longer going to allow the foods I eat to make me feel like a loser. From now on, I'm going to win with food.

Feel free to make a copy of this chapter, put a magnet on it, and hang it on your fridge, or reduce the size of the following pages and keep them in your purse or wallet for easy review.

As you read the following menus, check to see what you already have in your pantry or fridge. If you don't have them, put them on your shopping list. Are you ready here on Day 20 for some daily specifics on optimum health through better eating? If so, here we go . . .

SUNDAY

Breakfast

> Oat cereal (cooked with banana) or granola (avoid the heavily sugared brands)
> Skim or nonfat milk
> Unsweetened applesauce
> Herb tea

Mid-morning snack

> Fresh grapes

Lunch

> Black bean soup (use any recipe you can find, but hold off on the oil and salt) seasoned with lemon juice
> Tomato juice or fresh vegetable juice

Mid-afternoon snack

> Fresh orange

Dinner

> Succotash (lima beans and corn cooked with onions and spices). Think *variety!*
> Black-eyed peas flavored with onion
> Salad
> Pita bread
> Fresh fruit dessert

Breakfast

Oatmeal, granola, or yogurt (with "live cultures")
Ripe banana for sweetener (cook with oatmeal)
Nonfat milk
High-fiber, low-fat, whole grain toast
Herb tea

Mid-morning snack

Fresh apple (The fiber pectin in fresh fruits is extremely healthy. When you feel like reaching for something sugary in the morning, grab an apple. Your body will say thank-you.)

Lunch

Diversified salad (Vary the contents of your salads from meal to meal. Go for a rich variety of greens, fruits, and vegetables for lots of vitamins and minerals. Sorry, no avocado. These tasty delights are 75% fat and they just don't work with this permanent weight-loss program.)
Use lemon vinaigrette dressing or lemon wedges.

Mid-afternoon snack

Fresh pear

Dinner

Whole grain spaghetti or pasta (without egg)
Marinara sauce: Make with tomatoes, tomato paste (look for brands without salt), onion, garlic, mushrooms (they add both flavor and texture), bell peppers, and spices. Simmer for one hour without oil.
Diversified salad
Fresh fruit dessert

Breakfast

Buckwheat pancakes (Use egg whites instead of whole eggs in batter; add no butter or margarine. Spray skillet with Pam—it adds no calories.)

Unsweetened fruit spread for topping

Herb tea

Mid-morning snack

Two fresh plums (or be creative with any of your favorite fruits)

Lunch

Lentil soup (Fresh lentils, soaked and cooked with onions, carrots, herbs, and seasonings to taste, with no salt or oil. Use a thermos to carry to work. This will also keep you from caving in to your well-meaning but "pushy friends" who want you to gorge yourself at the all-you-can-eat trough.)

Diversified salad

Mid-afternoon snack

Fresh orange

Dinner

Stuffed bell pepper (Cooked bell peppers stuffed with steamed brown rice, tomatoes, fresh kernel corn, pimiento. Season with hot spices or a little stone-ground mustard. Isn't your mouth watering already?)

Diversified salad

Fresh fruit dessert

WEDNESDAY

Breakfast

Multigrain hot cereal
Banana, apricot, or raisins cooked in cereal for sweetener
Nonfat milk
Herb tea

Mid-morning snack

Fresh grapefruit sections (Yes, grapefruit is good at any time of the day—not just at breakfast.)

Lunch

Pita surprise (Whole grain pita or pocket bread, stuffed with sprouts, onions, tomatoes, parsley, cucumbers, seasoned with mustard. If you use a lot of stone-ground mustard, this healthy vegetable sandwich will taste like a hot dog! All you'll need is a ball game to go with it.)

Mid-afternoon snack

Fresh apple

Dinner

Steamed vegetables (carrots, broccoli, squash)
Steamed brown rice (herb and spice seasoning; no salt or oil)
Diversified salad
Fresh fruit dessert. Emphasis on *fresh*.

THURSDAY

Breakfast

Belgian waffles (1 cup whole wheat flour, 1 cup skim milk, 3 beaten egg whites; grease waffle iron with vegetable oil spray). Top with unsweetened fruit spread.
Herb tea

Mid-morning snack

Fresh fruit (This morning, try a fruit you've never had before! In fact, do this whenever you feel like it. The main thing is to eat FRUIT! Lots of it. Your insides will speak words of gratitude to you . . . pleading with you to continue to treat them with respect for many series of 21 days.)

Lunch

Vegetable soup (simmer vegetables with spices and herbs; no salt or oil)

Diversified salad

Mid-afternoon snack

Fresh grapes

Dinner

Baked potato

Homemade mock sour cream (nonfat yogurt with chives, chopped onions)

Kernel corn

Diversified salad

Fresh fruit dessert

FRIDAY

Breakfast

Puffed wheat or rice cereal with no preservatives

Fresh strawberries

Nonfat milk

Herb tea

Mid-morning snack

Fresh apple (By now, your body will be waiting for its mid-morning treat and will thank you forever for not giving it candy or packaged snack food.)

Lunch

Garbanzo inroad (Cooked garbanzo beans with onions and raw bell peppers. Mash until smooth; stuff into pocket bread with lettuce and tomato.)

Mid-afternoon snack

Fresh orange

Dinner

Chinese revelation (Steamed brown rice with Chinese vegetables: beans, sprouts, water chestnuts—good reason to go to a Chinese restaurant on occasion. I've found even if this is *not* on the menu, your Chinese server will more than likely be able to cook it up for you in no time.)
Season with Tamari sauce diluted half-and-half with water
Diversified salad
Fresh fruit dessert

SATURDAY

Breakfast

Cantaloupe (one-half)
Cracked whole wheat cereal cooked with banana
Nonfat milk
Herb tea

Mid-morning snack

Fresh grapefruit sections

Lunch

Homemade tomato soup (Use any cookbook recipe, but again, hold off on the oil and salt; season with herbs and spices.)

Mid-afternoon snack

Fresh pear

Dinner

Steamed garden diversified (steamed vegetables—carrots, corn, squash, bell peppers, mushrooms—seasoned with herbs and Pita bread or sourdough rye rolls)

Fresh fruit dessert

Now, I want you to review our menu again. Note the absence of such ingredients as caffeine, salad oils, and refined sugar. Even if you are unable to follow this suggested menu exactly, try to eat as many of these "kinds" of foods during the next 21 days—and beyond, and you'll be on your way to a life of exhilarating, permanent weight loss.

Now we've come to Day 21—one of the most exciting days of all the days we've been together . . . because what's coming up is the day you make the choice to turn your life around—for good! It's been a great journey together, so let's do it one more time.

LESSON OF THE DAY

I'm putting great food fuel in my tank;
I'm winning with food.

The Day You Turn Your Life Around

The Celebration Has Just Begun

Congratulations. You've made it to Day 21. As I read and reread the manuscript before I send it off to my publisher, I'm aware of the many things I've shared with you. One friend said, "Gregg, I couldn't do all that in 21 years!" He was kidding, of course. At least I *hope* he was. You see, you and I *can* do everything I've described in the previous 20 days. And we *can* make each of these principles "habits of the heart" as we make the sustained effort to think and eat better in the days, weeks, and years ahead.

Will it be easy? Not necessarily. Is there a possibility you might revert to some of your older, less-healthful eating habits? Yes, that's a distinct possibility. That's why I want you to read this book over and over. *Make your life a continual series of 21 days.* And, by the way, for those readers who already tend to be a bit obsessive-compulsive, don't *obsess* on the idea of 21 days. The important thing is to get on the program, and stay on the program, and forgive yourself if you fall away from the program, and then start anew. Keep at it, and you'll find your thinking patterns, and your eating habits, changing to the positive.

Now look at the title for today: *The Day You Turn Your Life Around*. This is the day. Day 21 is when you renew your commitment to taking such good care of your body that you will—from this day on—treat it with enormous respect, dignity, and the utmost of care. Welcome to the first really great day of the rest of your life.

AFFIRMATIONS FOR A LIFETIME

We've used many affirmations throughout these pages—positive words and statements I've asked you to repeat to yourself several times a day. Have you worked with these as we've gone along? Are you seeing and feeling the difference? In these closing pages, I want to give you 5 more *great food affirmations* to add to your collection. Try to say these at least 3 times a day—and repeat them with great emotion and enthusiasm:

1. Because I am eating better—and thinking about what I eat before I eat it—I have fewer illnesses, greater energy, reduced stress, and am recovering faster from any normal sickness.

2. I am enjoying my balanced diet. I feel great with my constant reduction of saturated fats. I love eating fruits and vegetables and am eating foods daily that help strengthen my immune system—compounds that include Vitamin C and beta-carotene.

3. I am enjoying regular, moderate exercising. I am increasing my blood flow and the oxygen to my brain, and I know this is accelerating the movement of immune cells around my body and is increasing the production of endorphins—my body's "feel-good" hormones.

4. God made my body as his temple, and I'm eating food with that in mind. I am eating for a healthy heart. I know that fruits and vegetables fight disease, and I am winning the battle against all illness. I am saying good-bye to too much sugar, fat, salt, and alcohol—all proven health risk factors.

5. I am a successful "smarter eating" tactician because I eat high-fiber foods such as beans, peas, whole grain cereals, and whole wheat pasta on a regular basis. Every day I eat foods to help me fight cancer, because I now know that when I take care of my body, my body will take care of me.

MY SUCCESS CHART

The above 5 affirmations will help remind you of the commitment to better eating you have made during these 21 days. With that in mind, I want you to take out a pencil and answer this question for each of the following important 6 categories—all areas we've explored in the past 3 weeks: *What am I doing well at the completion of my 21 days toward better eating?*

Emotionally I am

_____

In regard to physical exercise I am

_____

Nutritionally I am

_____

Relationally I am

_____

Spiritually I am

_____

In regard to affirmations I am

_____

JOURNAL YOUR PROGRESS

I encourage you to begin to journal your progress for the next three months. You may want to begin by expanding the use of your food journal to record your daily progress toward better eating habits in the above six areas. If you choose not to do this part of the assignment, I'm afraid you will not receive the full benefit of what you've just read and taken to heart. And I want the very best for you. So please begin your journal today.

If you've never journaled before—and you wonder if you really can do it—just think of journaling as writing a regular, affirming letter to yourself. Don't worry about spelling or grammar or sentence structure. The journal is *for your eyes only*. Just write down honest thoughts about where you are today, and, perhaps, an occasional comment on where you are planning to be six months, a year, or two years down the road. God may bring to mind a verse of Scripture that you'll want to record. Such verses may be the most rewarding part of your journaling experience. I want you to keep this personal record going for a minimum of three months. Over the years, I've discovered this one fact: *Only when we make the commitment to write down our feelings and thoughts will we be able to keep the change we desire alive and ongoing.* Here's how I would like you to conclude each journal entry. _____ (your name) remember . . . with God's help, *you have an exciting future and a life filled with hope!*

WHERE TO GO FROM HERE

I want to remind you that whoever you are, and wherever you are, the most important thing you can do—not only for the next 21 days but for the rest of your life—is to accept yourself as a beautiful, unrepeatable miracle from God. When you don't accept yourself, you run the risk of wasting your time looking for alternatives that, in the long run, will render you incomplete. *Accept yourself.* When you don't accept yourself, you will live in constant fear and dread of what each new day may hold for you. You no longer need to live that way. *Accept yourself.* When you don't accept yourself, you will always feel lonely, isolated, and out of touch, and you will tend to move toward food—and usually not the healthy variety—for your primary intimacy and comfort. Food is for nourishment, not a substitute for relationships. *Accept yourself.* Self-acceptance is not an unreachable goal but rather, a position from which you can choose to grow at any time in your life. Accept each part of yourself today, and what, for some reason, you cannot accept, be sure you quickly forgive.

It's been my pleasure to be your coach for these 21 days to better eating. Now, the fruit, vegetables, whole grain cereals, low-fat *everything*—and your new attitude toward the meaning of food—are in *your* shopping cart. Keep walking down the right aisles, knowing what's healthy and what's not. Keep asking yourself the key questions we've explored for the past 21 days. Continue saying your affirmations, aloud and with conviction. In the process, remember that you are a *whole person* and that life is so much more than just what you eat. That's why you need to keep yourself grounded in positive thinking about your better future. Because the *thinking* behind each of your actions is what will win the day for you as you make the daily decision to regard your body as a living temple of the living God. God bless you and keep you always—for all the many wonderful, exciting 21 days of your life that still lie ahead.

Bon appetit!

I would like to know something about your progress as you do this, so will you do me a favor? Drop me a line in three months or so. My address is:

Dr. Gregory L. Jantz,
The Center for Counseling and Health Resources, Inc.
611 Main Street
P.O. Box 700
Edmonds, WA 98020
drjantz
www.aplaceofhope.com
1-888-771-5166

I'm looking forward to hearing from you, and celebrating the success that I know will be yours.

LESSON OF THE DAY

Life is for Celebration . . . and I will
celebrate every one of the many exciting
"21 days of my life" still to come.

Look for all eight books in the 21-Day Series

The **21-Day Series** is perfect for anyone wanting to affect positive changes in their life. Studies have shown that virtually any habit can be established in a 21-day period. That's the idea behind the **21-Day Series**. If you are willing to concentrate on one important habit, using a day-by-day plan for change, then you can make positive, lasting improvements in your life.

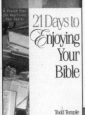

In *21 Days to Enjoying Your Bible*, youth leader and author Todd Temple shows you why the Bible is so fascinating, how to navigate its pages, how it is organized, and what personal, practical help the Bible offers. Softcover 0-310-21745-8

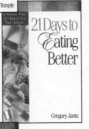

In *21 Days to Eating Better*, Gregory Jantz, who is founder and executive director of The Center for Counseling and Health Resources, uses proven strategies to teach you how to replace negative eating habits with energizing, healthy ways to feed and nurture not only the body but also your mind and soul.
Softcover 0-310-21747-4

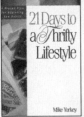

21 Days to a Thrifty Lifestyle by Mike Yorkey is all about spending money wisely, revealing practical ways to track expenses, how to save money, how to avoid being ripped off, and even includes plans for retirement, health care, and much more.
Softcover 0-310-21752-0

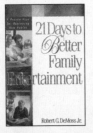

21 Days to Better Family Entertainment by youth culture expert Bob DeMoss supplies sensible advice to help families regain control of TV, music, movies, the Internet, and other forms of home entertainment. Here's a creative, realistic approach to trading media overload for a better family life. Softcover 0-310-21746-6

Available in April 1998:

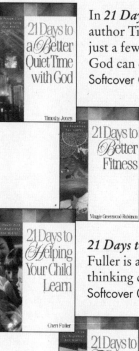

In *21 Days to a Better Quiet Time with God*, author Timothy Jones shows readers how taking just a few minutes from their day to share with God can enrich their lives immensely.
Softcover 0-310-21749-0

In *21 Days to Better Fitness*, leading health and fitness author Maggie Greenwood-Robinson offers readers a simple, day-by-day strategy for improving their fitness and health.
Softcover 0-310-21750-4

21 Days to Helping Your Child Learn by Cheri Fuller is a short course in teaching kids the joys of thinking creatively and learning naturally.
Softcover 0-310-21748-2

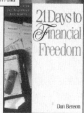

21 Days to Financial Freedom features a simple and practical financial plan that anyone can use, from the series' editor Dan Benson.
Softcover 0-310-21751-2

ZondervanPublishingHouse
Grand Rapids, Michigan
http://www.zondervan.com

We want to hear from you. Please send your comments about this book to us in care of the address below. Thank you.

ZondervanPublishingHouse
Grand Rapids, Michigan 49530
http://www.zondervan.com